START
SMART

FINISH
STRONG!

START SMART

FINISH STRONG!

Master the Fundamentals for Pain Free Fitness

KEVIN BROWN

gatekeeper press
rethink publishing

Prior to beginning any exercise program, you must consult with your physician. You must also consult your physician before increasing the intensity of your training.

Any application of the recommended material in this book is at the sole risk of the reader, and at the reader's discretion. Responsibility for any injuries or other adverse effects resulting from the application of information provided within this book is expressly disclaimed.

Published by Gatekeeper Press
3971 Hoover Rd. Suite 77
Columbus, OH 43123-2839
www.GatekeeperPress.com

ISBN: 9781619846296
eISBN: 9781619845961

Table of Contents

What is SMART Performance®?

INTRODUCTION

I am a physical therapist and fitness consultant. As a physical therapist, I treat musculoskeletal injuries and pain to help restore function. As a fitness consultant, I teach individuals how to maintain and improve physical health and how to safely achieve fitness goals. In both roles, my job involves evaluating movement and teaching exercise to improve health and function. Through my work as a physical therapist and fitness consultant I developed the **SMART Performance®** System.

SMART Performance® is a physical education system designed to teach fundamental exercises and movements for daily, recreational, and sporting activities. It provides a basic framework for individuals to develop and progress fitness programs that align with their specific goals. SMART is based on the practice and progression of fundamental movement and exercise skills. Learning and practicing these skills are the foundation of the **SMART Performance®** system, and are what enable individuals to safely improve their fitness level. My goal is to teach people how to master the movement and exercise skills necessary for them to maintain and improve their physical health.

Understanding how to use exercise to maintain and improve physical health is an invaluable skill for everyone to have. It will greatly increase your ability to prevent injury and continue living an active life even as you age. **SMART Performance®** provides you with a blueprint for how to effectively and efficiently use exercise to achieve lasting health and wellness.

HOW TO USE THIS BOOK

To best utilize this book, it's important to become familiarized with the foundations of **SMART Performance®**. Most of you will probably want to skip to the movement progressions, but don't do that. Understanding correct posture, alignment, and mechanics is a critical step to developing good movement. In the *Foundations of **SMART Performance®*** section, you'll discover how to assume and maintain correct posture, learn cues to maintain this posture through movements, gain a better understanding of how pain should guide your movements, and learn when to modify movements. After teaching the foundations of posture, alignment, and mechanics, I show you how to progress through the **SMART Performance®** system. In this section of the book, you will identify your current movement ability and individual movement needs through various exercises, stretches, and screenings. Findings generated from your assessment are used to create a personalized practice plan with a list of exercises that you should do. Mastery and maintenance of any skill, including movement, is achieved through consistent and proper practice, so embrace the journey to a STRONG finish.

I understand people have various fitness goals and achieving better fitness means different things to different people. With that in mind, I focused the content of this book on teaching fundamental exercise skills and concepts that are critical for everyone to have regardless of their fitness goals. It is meant to help people of any fitness level develop an individual practice plan that they can start with. However, once you progress through the **SMART Performance**® system, your path toward physical health and wellness will become more unique to fit your goals. To continue helping people reach their individual goals I created an online community. The community is focused on providing supportive content and answering specific questions from its members. To join the **SMART Performance**® community, visit us at smartperformanceconsultants.com. The **SMART Performance**® Community will be discussed further at the end of the book.

Foundations of SMART Performance®

PRINCIPLES

SMART represents the principles that guide our views of movement and exercise and their roles in establishing a solid foundation for both fitness and performance.

Safe: The movements and exercises practiced must always be within a person's ability level to ensure safety.

Mindful: The movements and exercises practiced require full mental engagement to be most effective.

Adaptive: The movements and exercises practiced reinforce the same foundational movement skills used for all forms of physical fitness and can easily be modified to meet an individual's specific needs

Repeatable: The movements and exercises practiced are best learned and mastered through repetition and proper practice

Therapeutic: The movements and exercises practiced help restore and maintain an individual's health and well-being and should not provoke pain.

MOVEMENT CONCEPTS

Pain = No gain:

Pain is a signal that something is wrong and should not be ignored. Trying to exercise through pain delays healing and can potentially make things worse. Pain alters movement and often causes compensatory movement patterns that can lead to further injury over time. If an exercise cause's pain, first make sure you are using proper form and mechanics. If correcting the form does not help, try modifying the movement or regressing the exercise. If you continue to have pain, then stop the exercise completely. After improving movement quality and strength with other exercises you should be able to perform the original exercise without pain.

If pain continues to be a limiting factor and does not allow you to perform fundamental movements it is important to be evaluated by a qualified medical professional. Pain that is present for a longer period of time is more difficult to treat so it is best to relieve symptoms and get improvement as quickly as possible.

Modify per mobility:

When people attempt to perform exercises that require an amount of mobility that they don't have, compensations occur and the risk of injury increases. When mobility is lacking the exercise needs to be modified to allow proper mechanics throughout the movement. If proper body mechanics cannot be maintained even with modifications, then the exercise should be stopped.

Prioritize your position:

When a person performs exercise with poor alignment, posture, or mechanics, it places them at increased risk for injury. Furthermore, when doing an exercise with poor form, the person will not get the desired benefit from that exercise. If good alignment, posture, or mechanics are not able to be achieved then the exercise needs to be modified or stopped completely.

POSTURE ALIGNMENT MECHANICS

At rest and during movement, good posture and alignment places the body in a better functional position. Having good posture is important because it allows the body to function as it was designed without placing abnormal stress on muscles and joints. Poor posture makes it more difficult to perform movements and places added stress on various areas of the body. Over time, this can lead to injury, pain, and decreased function.

To achieve better posture:

— Try to be more aware of your body's position during the day and make an effort to correct your posture when you notice a bad position.
— Avoid sitting or standing in one position for too long. If you sit a lot during the day, try to get up or change positions more often.
— Maintain and develop good postural mobility and strength with regular exercise.

Achieving good posture requires adequate mobility and proper muscle activation of postural muscles. Postural muscles are meant to be active and engaged during the majority of all movement and activity. They include short neck flexors, scapular stabilizers, and core and glut muscles

Poor posture occurs when the head and neck are forward, the shoulders are rounded, or the low back is slumped causing the pelvis to have an increased posterior tilt. In these positions the short neck flexors and scapular stabilizers are not engaged and the neck extensors and anterior chest muscles are in a shortened position. Additionally, the low back is placed in a vulnerable position

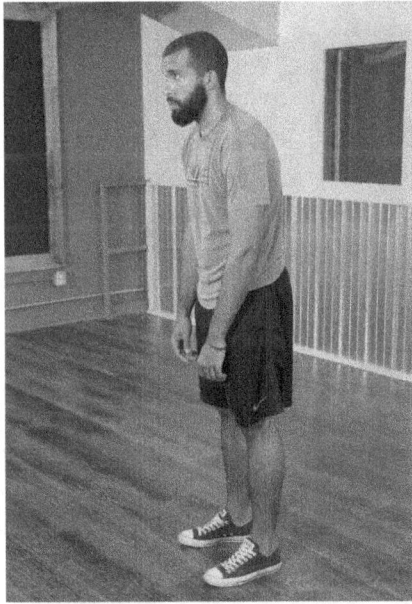

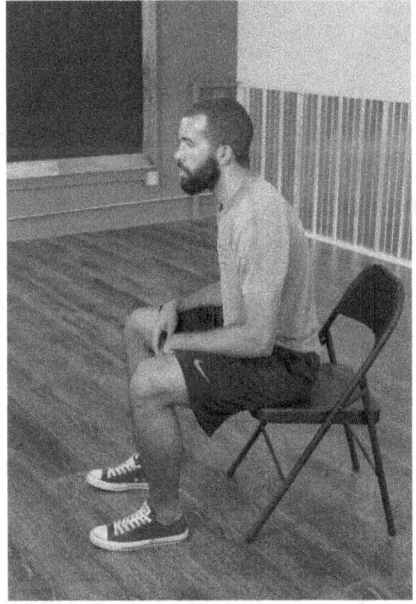

Poor Standing Posture
Forward head, rounded shoulders, and slumped low back/increased posterior pelvic tilt.

Poor Sitting Posture
Forward head, rounded shoulders, and slumped low back/increased posterior pelvic tilt.

Poor posture also occurs when the low back is overextended, causing the pelvis to have an increased anterior tilt. In this position, the core is not engaged and the hip flexors and low back extensors are in a shortened position.

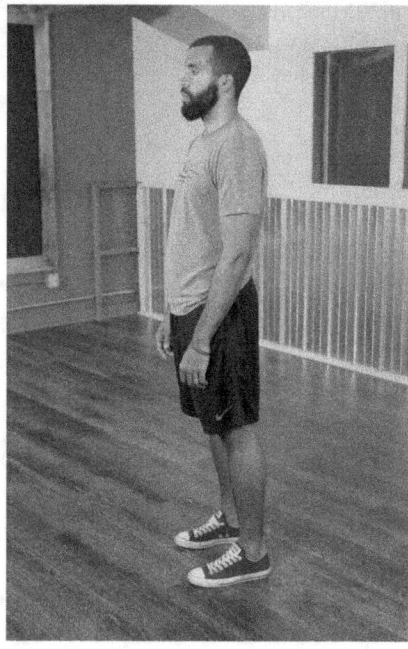

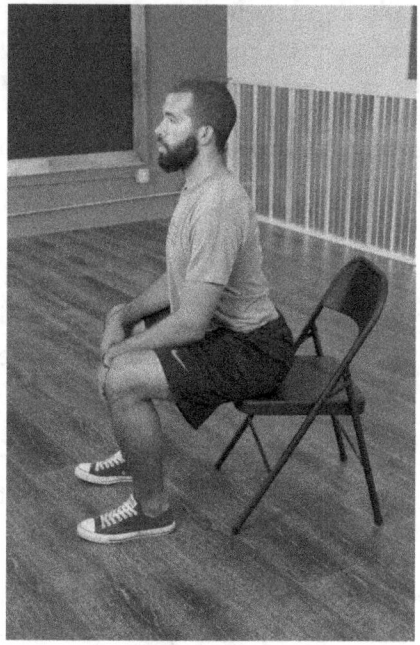

Poor Standing Posture
Excessive low back arch/increased anterior pelvic tilt.

Poor Sitting Posture
Excessive low back arch/increased anterior pelvic tilt.

Good posture occurs when the ears, shoulders and hips are in alignment. Good posture is achieved by performing a subtle chin tuck motion, slightly pulling the shoulders back and down, and engaging the core and gluts. This activates the short neck flexors and scapular stabilizers and places the low back and pelvis in a neutral position. The neutral position for the low back has a slight inward curve.

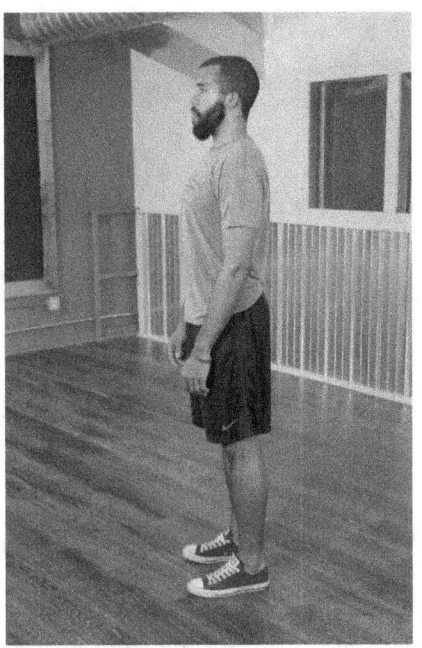

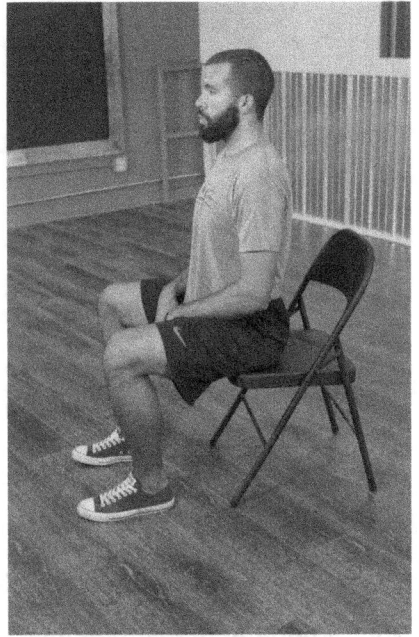

Good Standing Posture
Ears, shoulders, and hips are aligned; neutral spine and pelvis with postural muscles engaged.

Good Sitting Posture
Ears, shoulders, and hips are aligned; neutral spine and pelvis with postural muscles engaged.

Things to look for when assessing standing and sitting posture:

- Are the ears in line with the shoulders and are the short neck flexors engaged to maintain the position?
- Are the shoulder blades engaged to properly align the shoulders or are the shoulders rounded and forward?
- Is the low back and pelvis in a neutral position or is there an increased arch or rounding in the low back?
- Are the rib cage and abdominals pulled in and down or is the stomach puffed out?

Other components of proper upright posture, alignment and lifting/bending mechanics:

In the standing position, the knees should be in what is called a relaxed stance. They are straight but not locked out or hyperextended. When bending the knees, bending down to lift something, or loading the lower body, the weight should be absorbed through the hips. This occurs by sitting the butt back and hinging at the hips while maintaining a neutral spine and engaged core. This prevents the knees from going forward over the toes or collapsing inward and protects the spine when bending. The knees going forward or collapsing inward or the low back losing neutral spine is a sign of poor mechanics.

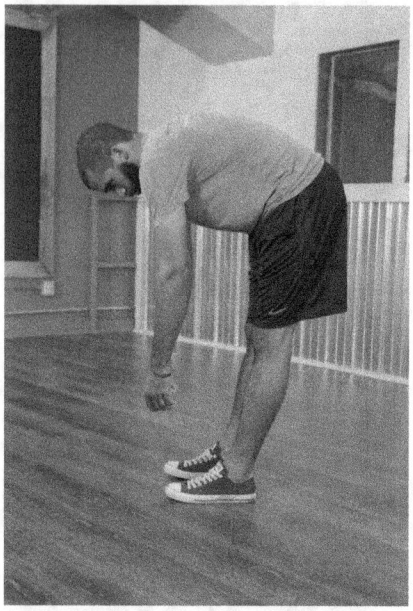

Poor lifting/bending mechanics
Rounded/flexed low back.

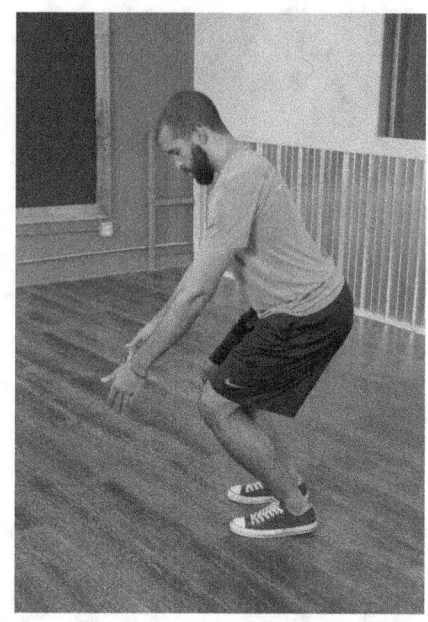

Poor lifting/bending mechanics
No posterior weight shift; forward
knee position.

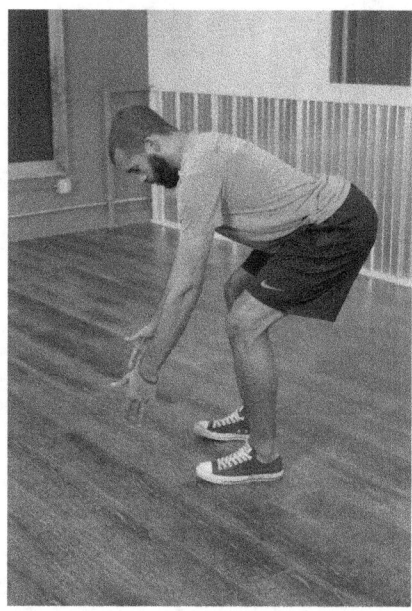

**Proper lifting/bending
mechanics**

Neutral spine; posterior weight
shift/hips shifted backward;
vertical knee position.

SMART Performance® System

SYSTEM OVERVIEW

1. Breathing and Core Engagement
2. Foundational Exercises
3. Postural and Upper Body Exercises
4. Mobility and Stretching
5. Screening for Running and Jumping

UNDERSTANDING THE SYSTEM

Ideal Ability (IA): This means you are able to perform the exercise with perfect form while showing ideal foundational ability in terms of endurance and strength for that particular exercise. The exercise is appropriate for you to perform and you are able to safely progress the exercise.

Perfect Form (PF): This means you are able to perform the exercise with perfect form based on the criteria given but lack foundational strength or endurance for that particular exercise. (Example: You can perform five pushups in a row with perfect form but are unable to do a set of twenty.) The exercise is appropriate for you to perform and you should work toward achieving ideal ability.

Appropriate to Perform (AP): This means you have enough ability to perform the exercise safely but certain aspects of the movement could be improved. The exercise is appropriate for you to perform. You should continue performing the exercise while working to improve form and ability. Also, perform any appropriate corrective exercises and stretches that will help improve the movement.

Not Appropriate to Perform (NA): This means the exercise is not safe for you to perform or would not be a beneficial exercise for you to perform right now. You should perform the next exercise in the progression along with any of the appropriate corrective exercises and stretches that could help improve quality and teach the movement.

APPLYING THE SYSTEM

Breathing and Engaging the Core

Prior to performing any exercises, you must understand how to breathe correctly and properly engage the core in all positions.

Often when learning how to breathe properly and engage the core it is easiest to first practice lying on your back in the supine position, then transition the skill to standing and other positions.

Steps for learning proper breathing and core engagement:

1. Learn proper breathing in supine.
2. Learn how to engage the core and breathe in supine with both knees bent and knees straight.
3. Transition proper breathing and core engagement/neutral spine to standing and other positions.

How to perform supine breathing:

Lie on your back with the knees bent up and breathe in through the nose and out through the mouth. Place one hand on the stomach so you can feel the movement of the stomach with the breath.

Additional information:

The belly should rise on the inhale and fall during the exhale without the chest and shoulders being elevated. On the exhale, the rib cage and abdominals should naturally be pulled in and down toward the spine causing the abdominals to tighten slightly.

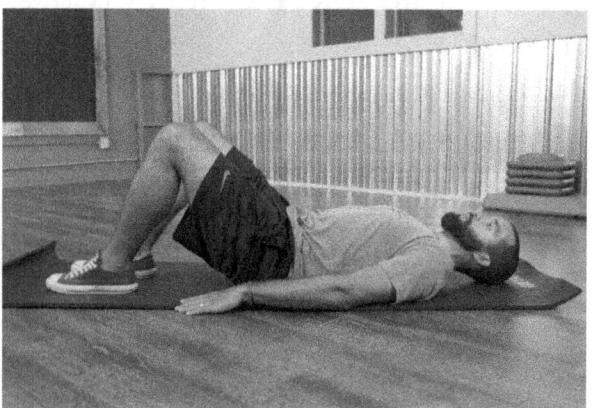

Proper breathing mechanics:
Stomach rises during inhale and falls during exhale.

How to engage the core and achieve neutral spine in supine with knees bent:

Lie on your back with the knees bent up, flatten the low back to the ground, and tighten the abdominals. The rib cage and abdominal should be pulled in and down toward the spine. You can place your hand or a small towel under the back to cue yourself to flatten the low back. With the core engaged, perform proper breathing.

Additional information:

To flatten the low back to the ground, you can also think about slightly rotating the pelvis backward to a neutral position. With the knees bent up the pelvis is biased toward a neutral position so the amount of posterior pelvic tilt should be minimal. With the core engaged, perform proper breathing.

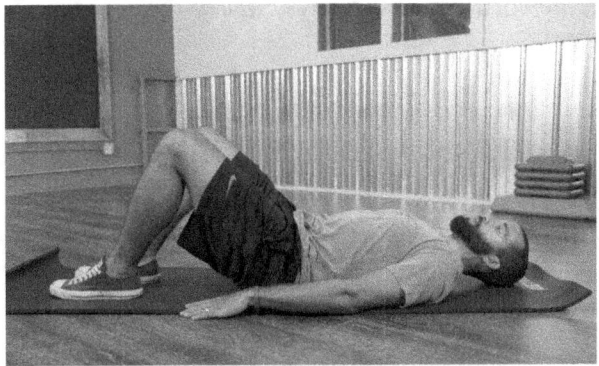

Engaging the core with knees bent:
Low back is flat to the ground; abdominals are tightened.

How to engage the core and achieve neutral spine in supine with knees straight:

Lie on your back with the knees straight and squeeze the gluts, flatten the low back to the ground, and lightly tighten the abdominals. The rib cage and abdominals should be pulled in down toward the spine. With the core engaged, perform proper breathing.

Additional information:

To flatten the low back to the ground, you can also think about rotating the pelvis backward to a neutral position but for most people squeezing the gluts and tightening the abdominals naturally places the pelvis in a neutral position. With the core engaged, perform proper breathing.

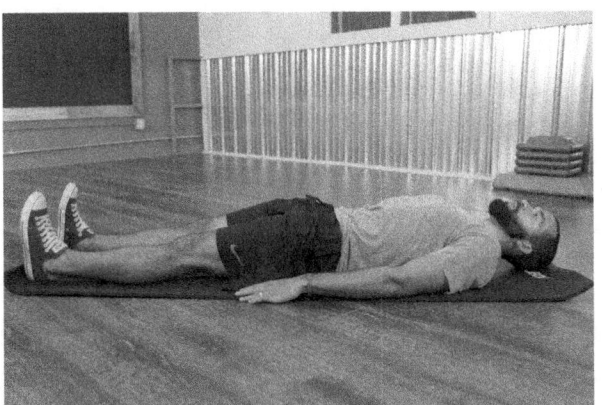

Engaging the core with knees straight:
Low back is flat to the ground; abdominals are tightened.

When you understand how to breathe correctly and engage the core in the supine position, practice it standing using the same mechanics. While performing any exercise, you need to be able to breathe correctly and engage the core in order to perform the exercise safely.

Things to look for when learning proper breathing and core engagement in the supine position:

— Is the back flat to the floor?
— Are the rib cage and abdominals pulled in and down or is the stomach puffed out?
— Is the pelvis neutral or is there too much tilt causing the hips to come off the ground?
— Does breathing occur through the stomach or are the chest and shoulders moving up and down as well?
— Can you engage the core and breathe correctly at the same time without excessive effort?

Foundational Exercises

1. Reverse Active Straight Leg Raise
2. Double Leg Lowering
3. Single Leg/Double Leg Bridge
4. Bird Dog UE/LE
5. Plank
6. Side Plank
7. Push Up
8. Double Leg and Single Leg RDL
9. Step Back Lunge
10. Body Weight Squat

REVERSE ASLR PROGRESSION

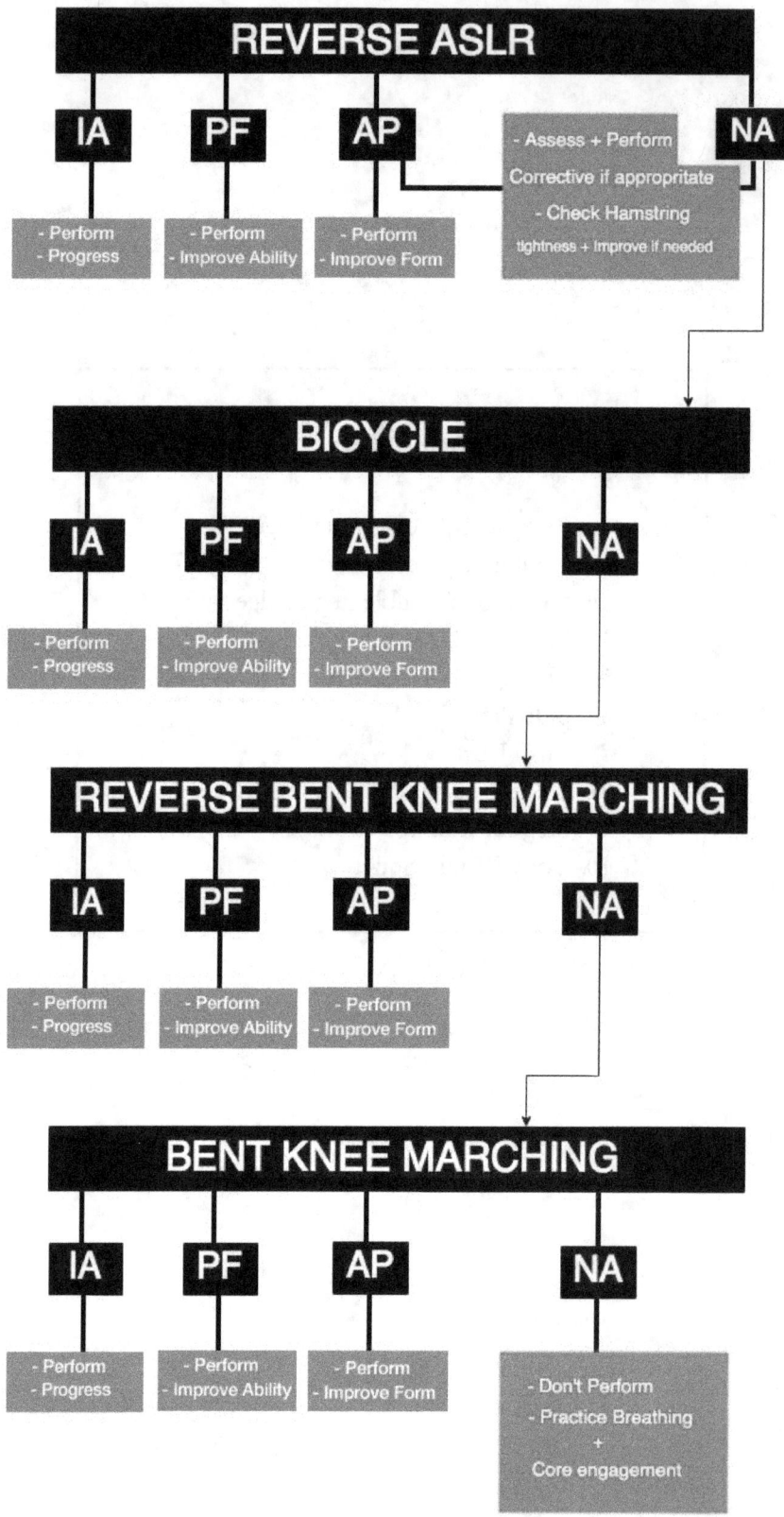

Reverse Active Straight Leg Raise (ASLR)

How to perform: Lie on your back with the hips flexed to 90 degrees and knees straight, pointing the feet up at the ceiling. Engage the core and lower one leg, tapping the heel to the floor and lift back up. Alternate between sides.

Additional information: Keep the head and low back flat to the floor throughout. Keep both knees straight and don't let the feet turn out.

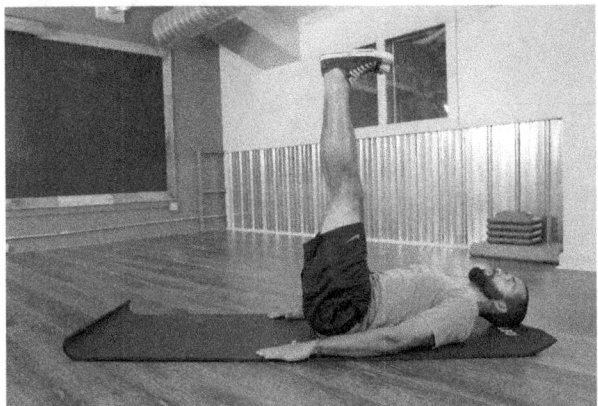

(a) Lie on your back with feet pointing straight up;

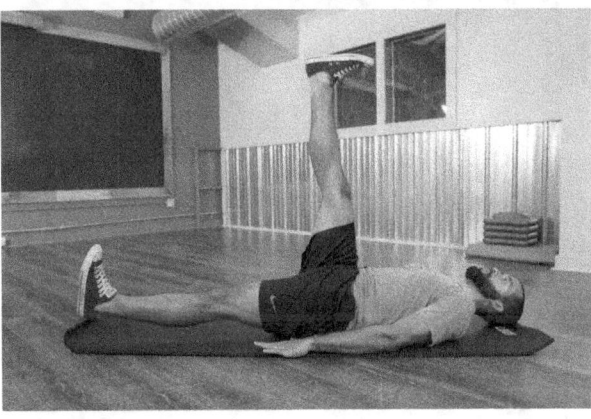

(b) Lower the leg.

Ideal ability: Able to complete a set of 20 repetitions alternating between right and left with perfect form and minimal difficulty.

Perfect form includes: No loss of neutral spine/core engagement (back stays flat and rib cage doesn't flair out). The knees stay straight throughout. Able to lower the right and left leg all the way to the ground and lift back up.

Not appropriate to perform if: Unable to maintain neutral spine/core engagement (back comes off ground or rib cage flairs out), or if movement causes pain.

If the reverse ASLR exercise is appropriate to perform but form requires improvement, continue performing the reverse ASLR exercise while working to improve form. Perform ASLR corrective if appropriate. Check hamstring mobility and, if limited, work to improve it (see *Mobility and Stretching* section for how to assess and improve hamstring mobility).

If the reverse ASLR exercise is inappropriate to perform, assess if the bicycle exercise is appropriate to perform. Perform ASLR corrective if appropriate. Check hamstring mobility and, if limited, work to improve it (see *Mobility and Stretching* section for how to assess and improve hamstring mobility).

How to progress or make harder: Perform the reverse ASLR exercise with arms over head.

Reverse Active Straight Leg Raise Corrective

How to perform: Lie on your back next to a doorway and flex both hips to 90 degrees with the knees straight, pointing the feet up at the ceiling (one leg will rest on the wall). Engage the core and lower the unsupported leg, tapping the heel to the floor and lift back up. Perform the exercise on both sides.

Additional information: Keep the head and low back flat to the floor throughout. Keep both knees straight and don't let the feet turn out.

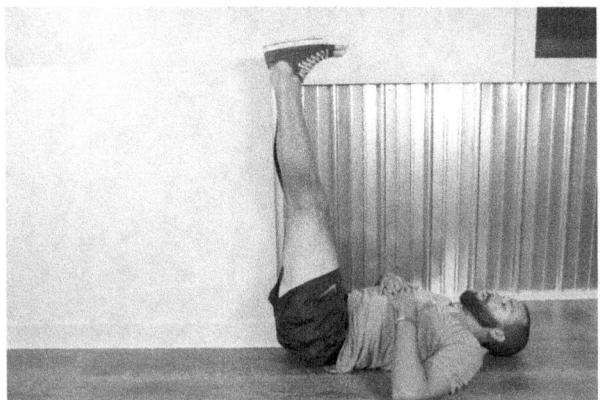

(a) Lie on your back in a doorway with feet pointing straight up;

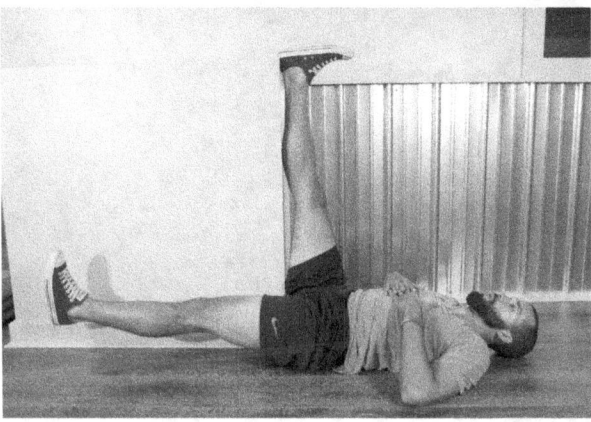

(b) Lower the unsupported leg.

Perfect form includes: No loss of neutral spine/core engagement (back stays flat and rib cage doesn't flair out). Keep the knees straight throughout. Ability to lower the right and left leg all the way to the ground and lift back up.

Not appropriate to perform if: Unable to maintain neutral spine/core engagement (back comes off ground or rib cage flairs out) or causes pain.

If the ASLR corrective is appropriate to perform but form requires improvement, continue performing the ALSR corrective while working to improve form.

If the ASLR corrective is not appropriate to perform, hold off on the ASLR corrective.

Bicycle

How to perform: Lie on your back with the knees and hips flexed to 90 degrees. Engage the core and extend one leg straight out and lower it, tapping the heel to the floor and lift back up. Alternate between left and right legs.

Additional information: Keep the head and low back flat to the floor throughout.

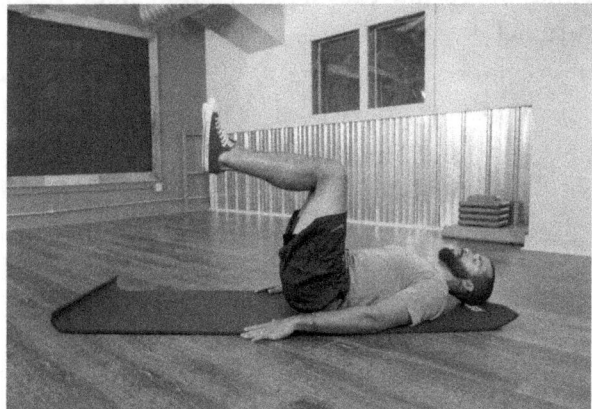

(a) Lie on your back with hips flexed and knees bent;

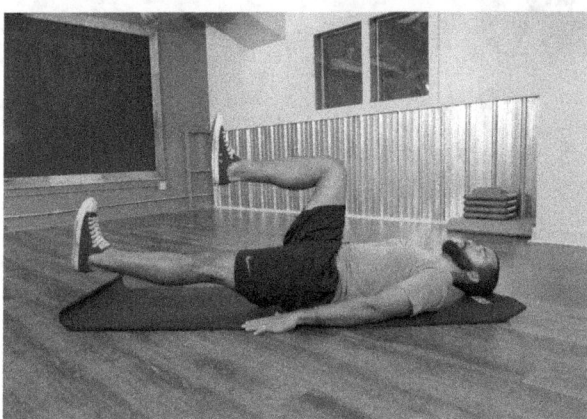

(b) Extend the knee and lower the leg.

Ideal ability: Able to complete a set of 20 repetitions alternating between right and left with perfect form and minimal difficulty.

Perfect form includes: No loss of neutral spine/core engagement (back stays flat and rib cage doesn't flair out). Able to lower the right and left leg all the way to the ground and lift back up.

Not appropriate to perform if: Unable to maintain neutral spine/core engagement (back comes off ground or rib cage flairs out), or if movement causes pain.

If the bicycle exercise is appropriate to perform but form requires improvement, continue performing the bicycle exercise while working to improve form.

If the bicycle exercise is not appropriate to perform, assess if the reverse bent knee marching exercise is appropriate to perform.

How to progress or make harder: Perform the bicycle exercise with arms over head.

Reverse Bent Knee Marching

How to perform: Lie on your back with the knees and hips flexed to 90 degrees. Engage the core and lower one leg, tapping the heel to the floor and lift back up. Alternate between left and right legs.

Additional information: Keep the head and low back flat to the floor throughout. When lowering the leg, extend the hip and keep both knees bent at 90 degrees throughout.

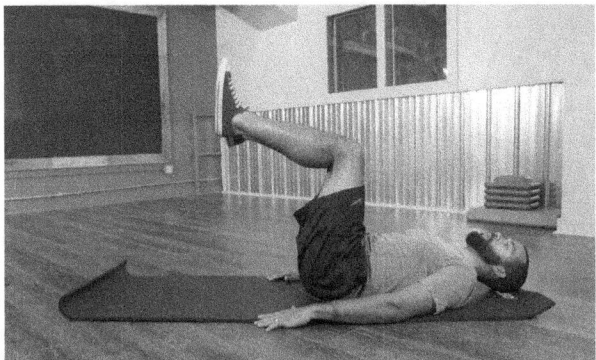

(a) Lie on your back with hips flexed and knees bent;

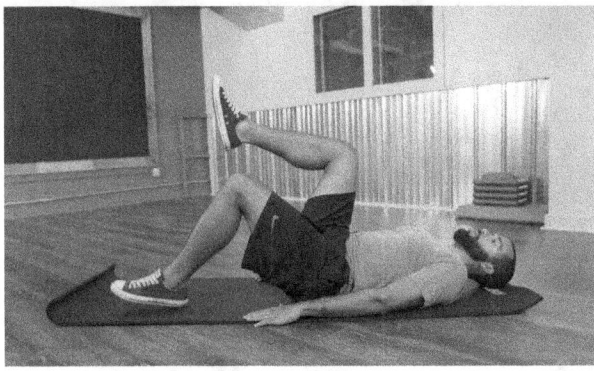

(b) Lower the leg.

Ideal ability: Able to complete a set of 20 repetitions alternating between right and left with perfect form and minimal difficulty.

Perfect form includes: No loss of neutral spine/core engagement (back stays flat and rib cage doesn't flair out). Able to lower the right and left leg all the way to the ground and lift back up.

Not appropriate to perform if: Unable to maintain neutral spine/core engagement (back comes off ground or rib cage flairs out), or if movement causes pain.

If the reverse bent knee marching exercise is appropriate to perform but form requires improvement, continue performing the reverse bent knee marching exercise and work to improve form.

If the reverse bent knee marching exercise is not appropriate to perform, assess if the bent knee marching exercise is appropriate to perform.

How to progress or make harder: Perform the reverse bent knee marching exercise with arms over head.

Bent Knee Marching

How to perform: Lie on your back with knees bent up. Engage the core and lift one knee up to 90 degrees and lower back down; alternate between left and right legs.

Additional information: Keep the head and low back flat to the floor.

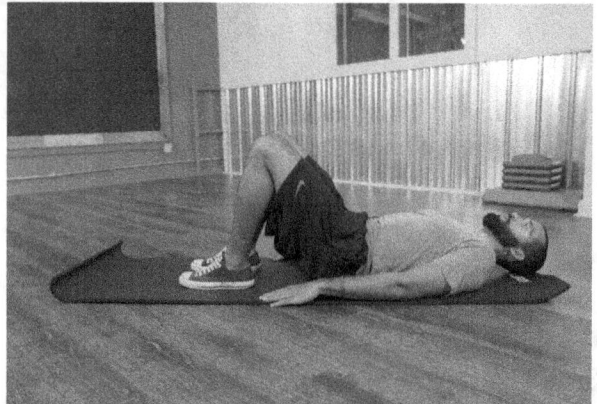

(a) Lie on your back with knees bent up;

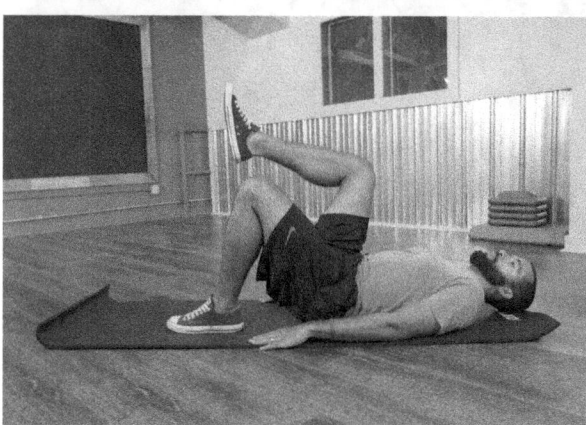

(b) Lift the knee up.

Ideal ability: Able to perform a set of 20 repetitions alternating between right and left with perfect form and minimal difficulty.

Perfect form includes: No loss of neutral spine/core engagement (back stays flat and rib cage doesn't flair out) and able to lift the right and left knee up to 90 degrees and low back down with control.

Not appropriate to perform if: Unable to maintain neutral spine/core engagement (back comes off ground or rib cage flairs out), or movement causes pain.

If the bent knee marching exercise is appropriate to perform but form requires improvement, continue performing the bent knee marching exercise while working to improve form.

If the bent knee marching exercise is inappropriate to perform, work on engaging the core and proper breathing.

How to progress and make harder: Perform the bent knee marching exercise with arms overhead.

DOUBLE LEG LOWER PROGRESSION

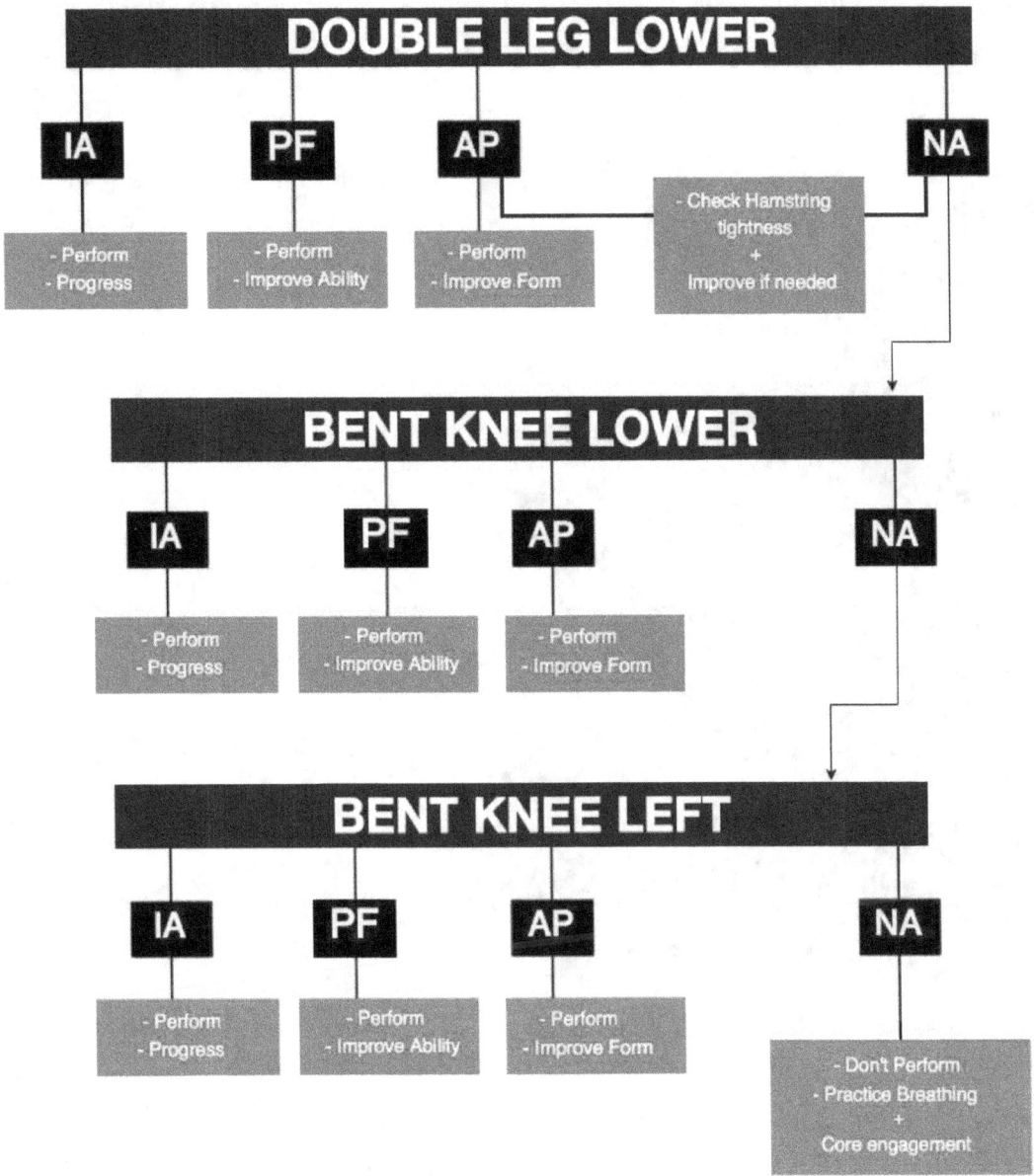

Double Leg Lowering

How to perform: Lie on your back with the hips flexed to 90 degrees and knees straight, pointing the feet up at the ceiling. Engage the core and lower both legs tapping the heels to the floor and lift back up.

Additional information: Keep the head and low back flat to the floor throughout. Keep the legs straight.

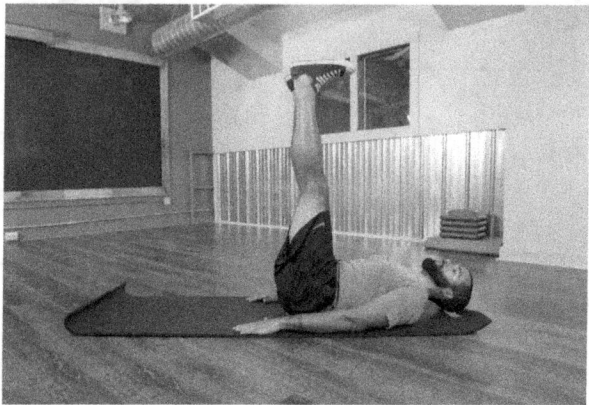

(a) Lie on your back with feet pointing straight up;

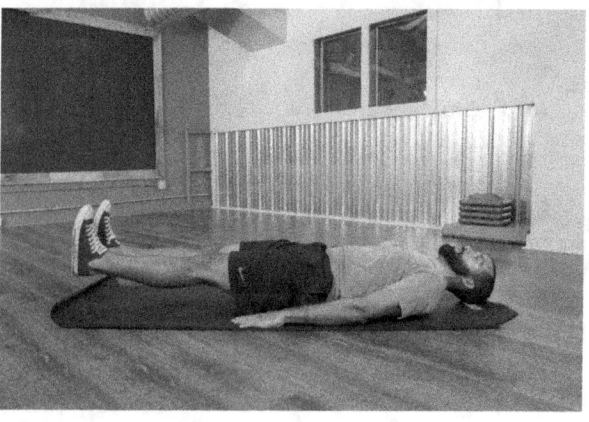

(b) Lower the legs.

Ideal ability: Able to perform a set of 20 repetitions with perfect form and minimal difficulty.

Perfect form includes: No loss of neutral spine/core engagement (back stays flat and rib cage doesn't flair out). The knees stay straight throughout. Ability to lower the legs all the way to the ground and lift back up.

Not appropriate to perform if: Unable to maintain neutral spine/core engagement (back comes off ground or rib cage flairs out) or if movement causes pain.

If the double leg lowering exercise is appropriate to perform but form requires improvement, continue performing the double leg lowering exercise while working to improve form. Check hamstring mobility and, if limited, work to improve it (see *Mobility and Stretching* section for how to assess and improve hamstring mobility).

If the double leg lowering exercise is inappropriate to perform: Assess if the reverse bent knee lowering exercise is appropriate to perform. Check hamstring mobility and, if limited, work to improve it (see *Mobility and Stretching* section for how to assess and improve hamstring mobility).

How to progress double leg lowering or make harder: Perform the double leg lowering exercise with arms over head.

Bent Knee Lowering

How to perform: Lie on your back with the knees and hips flexed to 90 degrees. Engage the core and lower both legs, tapping the heels to the floor and lift back up.

Additional information: Keep the head and low back flat to the floor.

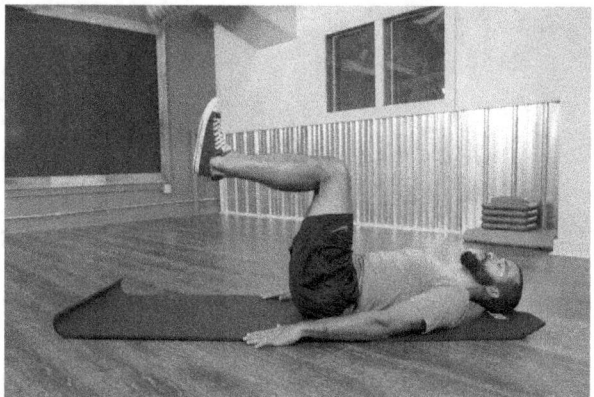

(a) Lie on your back with hips flexed and knees bent;

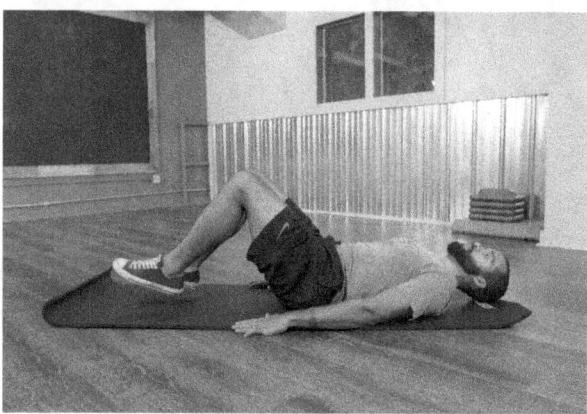

(b) Lower the legs.

Ideal ability: Able to perform a set of 20 repetitions with perfect form and minimal difficulty.

Perfect form includes: No loss of neutral spine/core engagement (back stays flat and rib cage doesn't flair out), and able to lower the legs all the way to the ground and lift back up.

Not appropriate to perform if: Unable to maintain neutral spine/core engagement (back comes off ground or rib cage flairs out) or causes pain.

If the bent knee lowering exercise is appropriate to perform but form requires improvement, continue performing the bent knee lowering exercise while working to improve form.

If the bent knee lowering exercise is inappropriate to perform, assess if the bent knee lift exercise is appropriate to perform.

How to progress bent knee lowering or make harder: Perform the bent knee lowering exercise with arms overhead.

Bent Knee Lift

How to perform: Lie on your back with the knees bent up. Engage the core and flex both knees up to 90 degrees and lower back down.

Additional information: Keep the head and low back flat to the floor.

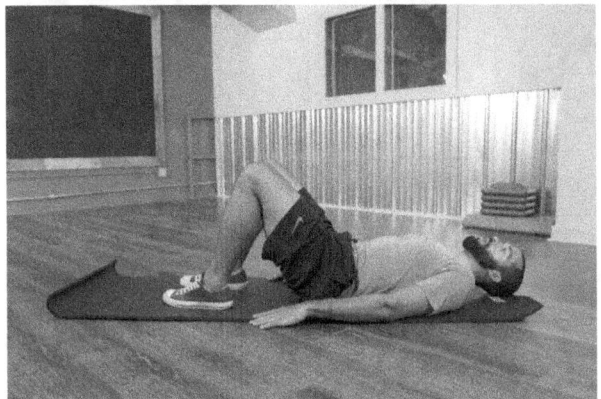

(a) Lie on your back with knees bent up;

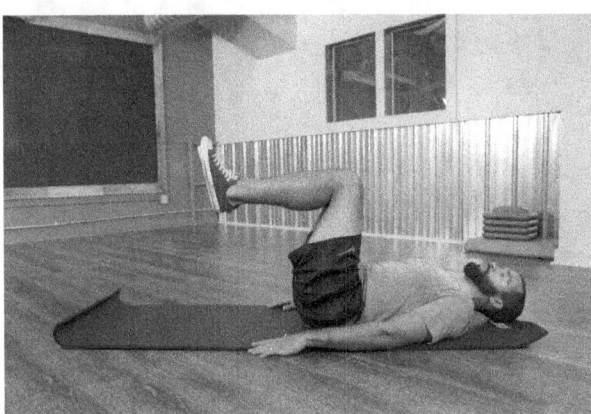

(b) Lift the legs.

Ideal ability: Able to perform a set of 20 repetitions with perfect form and minimal difficulty.

Perfect form Includes: No loss of neutral spine/core engagement (back stays flat and rib cage doesn't flair out) and able to lift knees up to 90 degrees and lower back down with control.

Not appropriate to perform if: Unable to maintain neutral spine/core engagement (back comes off ground or rib cage flairs out) or if movement causes pain.

If the bent knee lift exercise is appropriate to perform but form requires improvement, continue performing the bent knee lift exercise while working to improve quality.

If the bent knee lift exercise is inappropriate to perform, work on engaging the core in supine and proper breathing.

How to progress or make harder: Perform the bent knee lift exercise with arms over head.

SINGLE LEG BRIDGE PROGRESSION

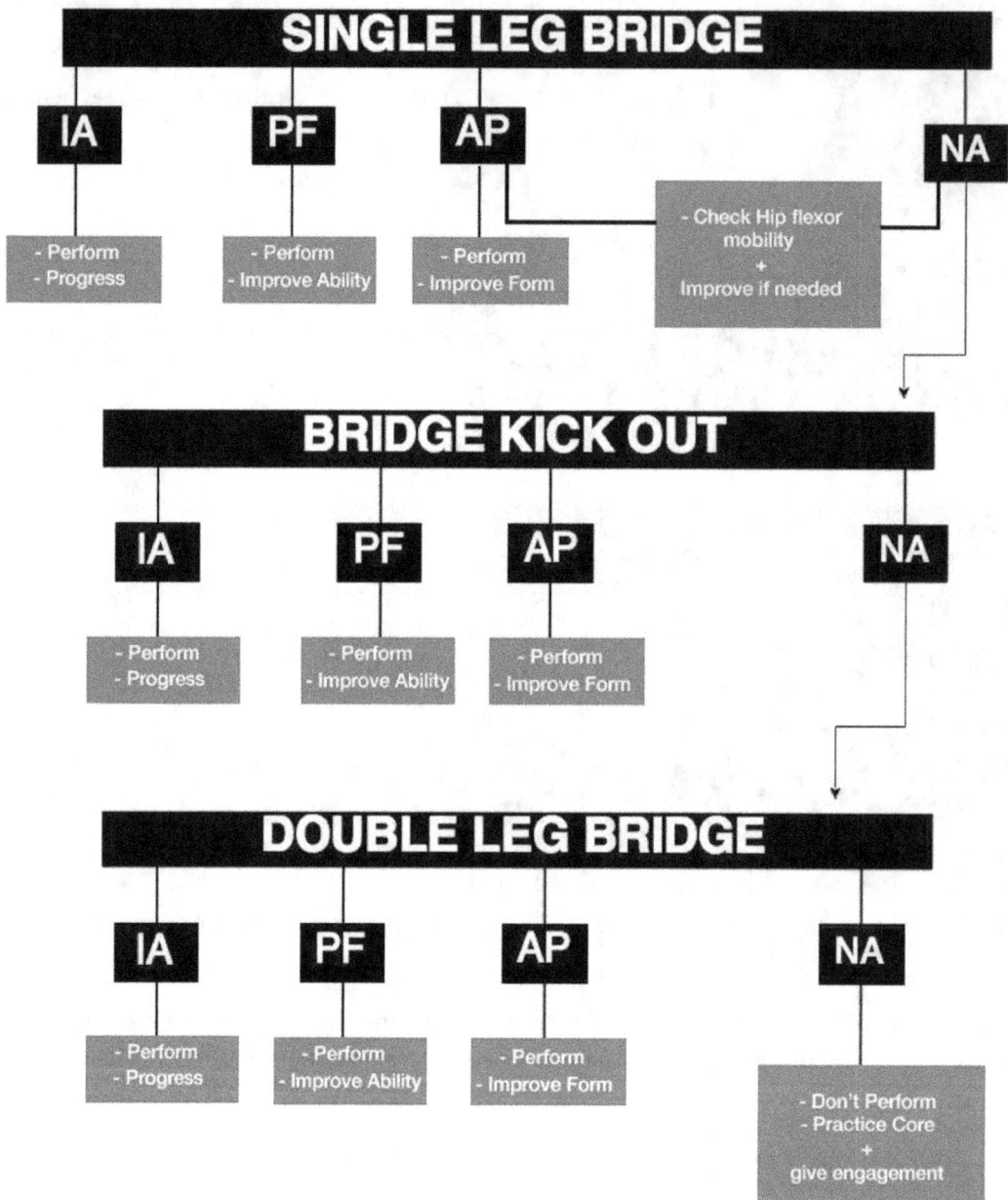

SINGLE LEG BRIDGE

IA
- Perform
- Progress

PF
- Perform
- Improve Ability

AP
- Perform
- Improve Form

NA
- Check Hip flexor mobility
+
Improve if needed

BRIDGE KICK OUT

IA
- Perform
- Progress

PF
- Perform
- Improve Ability

AP
- Perform
- Improve Form

NA

DOUBLE LEG BRIDGE

IA
- Perform
- Progress

PF
- Perform
- Improve Ability

AP
- Perform
- Improve Form

NA
- Don't Perform
- Practice Core
+
give engagement

Single Leg Bridge

How to perform: Lie on your back with one knee bent up and the other leg extended pointed at the ceiling. Engage the core, squeeze the gluts, and extend the hip, lifting the butt off the floor. Pause 1 to 2 seconds and lower back down.

Additional information: Keep the head flat to the floor and maintain a neutral spine throughout. Don't arch the low back. The majority of tension should be felt in the gluts without experiencing hamstring cramping or low back tightness.

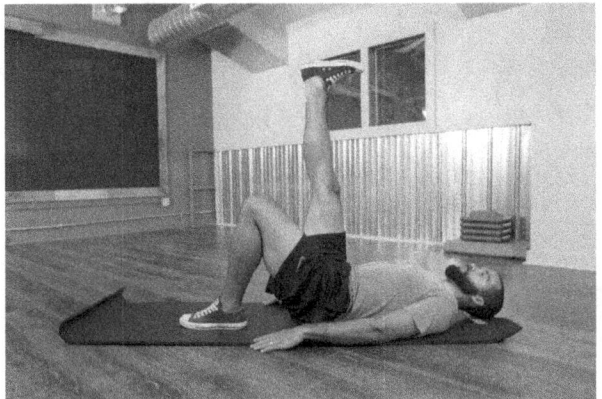

(a) Lie on your back with one knee bent up and one leg pointing straight up;

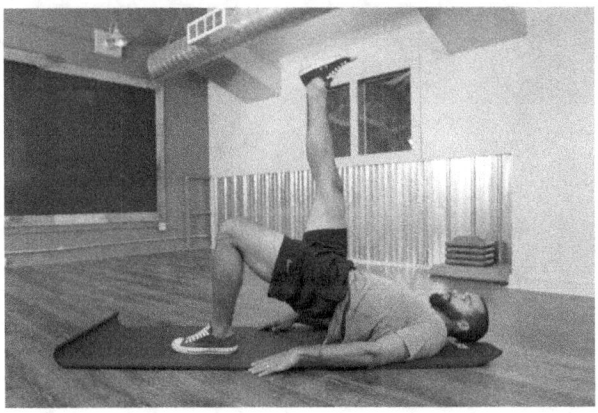

(b) Lift the butt off the floor.

Ideal ability: Able to perform a set of 20 repetitions on the right and left with perfect form and minimal difficulty.

Perfect form includes: Able to achieve full hip extension. No loss of neutral spine/core engagement (The low back doesn't arch and ribs don't flair out). Pelvis remains level. No hamstring cramping or low back tightness.

Not appropriate to perform if: Unable to lift the butt off the floor; unable to maintain a neutral spine (back arches or ribs flair out), or if movement causes pain.

If the single leg bridge exercise is appropriate to perform but form requires improvement, continue performing the single leg bridge exercise while working to improve form. Check hip flexor mobility and if limited work to improve it (see *Mobility and Stretching* section for how to assess and improve hip flexor mobility).

If the single leg bridge exercise is inappropriate to perform, assess if the bridge kick out exercise is appropriate to perform. Check hip flexor mobility and if limited work to improve it (see *Mobility and Stretching* section for how to assess and improve hip flexor mobility).

Bridge Kick Out

How to perform: Lie on your back with the knees bent up. Engage the core, squeeze the gluts, then extend the hips, lifting the butt off the floor. When the hips are fully extended, kick one leg out; hold for 5 seconds and lower back down.

Additional information: Keep the head flat on the floor and maintain a neutral spine throughout, don't arch the low back. The majority of tension should be felt in the gluts without experiencing hamstring cramping or low back tightness.

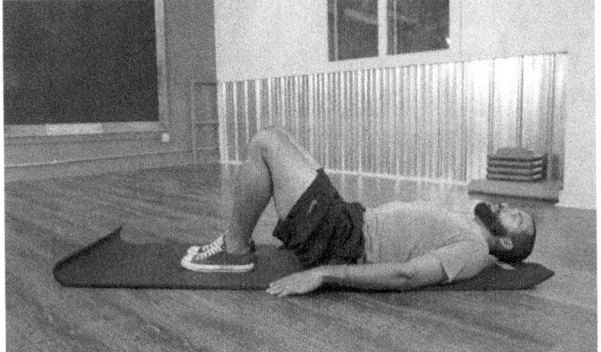

(a) Lie on your back with knees bent up;

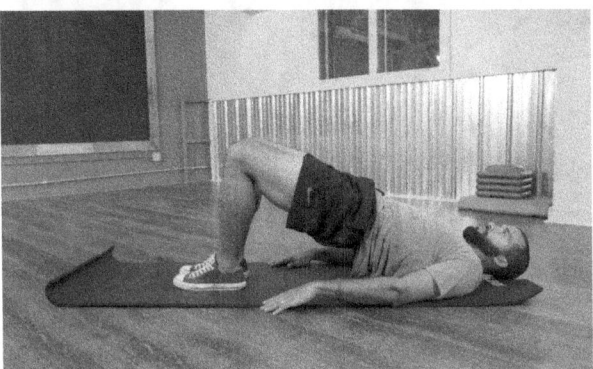

(b) Lift the butt off the floor;

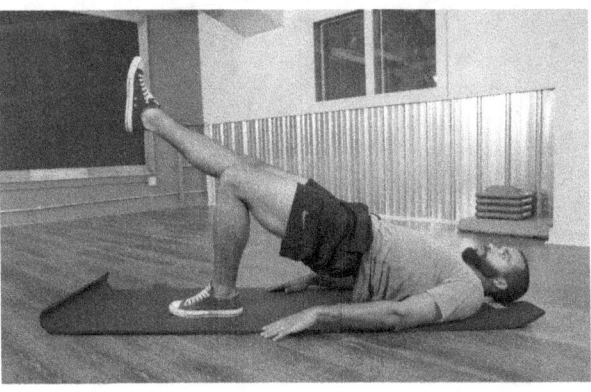

(c) Kick the leg straight out.

Ideal ability: Able to perform a set of 10 repetitions on the right and left with perfect form and minimal difficulty.

Perfect form includes: Able to achieve full hip extension. No loss of neutral spine/core engagement (low back doesn't arch or and ribs don't flair out). Able to hold for 5 seconds and maintain a level pelvis throughout. No hamstring cramping or low back tightness.

Not appropriate to perform if: Unable to lift the butt off the floor; unable to extend leg and maintain balance and control for at least 1 second; unable to maintain a neutral spine (back arches or ribs flair out), or movement causes pain.

If the single leg bridge kick out exercise is appropriate to perform but the form requires improvement, continue performing the single leg bridge kick out exercise out while working to improve form.

If the single leg bridge kick out exercise out is inappropriate to perform, assess if the double leg bridge exercise is appropriate to perform.

Double Leg Bridge

How to perform: Lie on your back with the knees bent up. Engage the core. Squeeze the gluts, then extend the hips, lifting the butt off the floor. Pause 1 to 2 seconds and lower back down.

Additional information: Keep the head flat to the floor and maintain a neutral spine throughout; don't arch the low back. The majority of tension should be felt in the gluts without experiencing hamstring cramping or low back tightness.

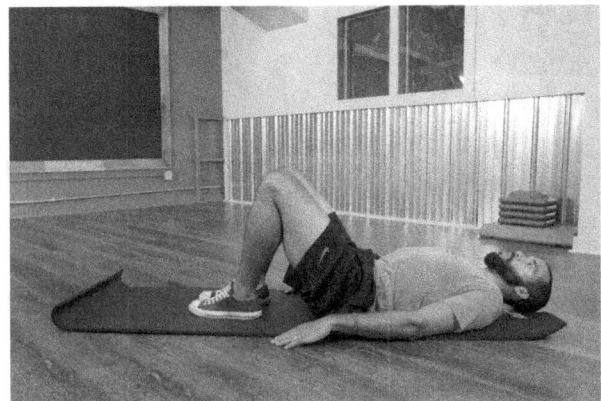

(a) Lie on your back with knees bent up;

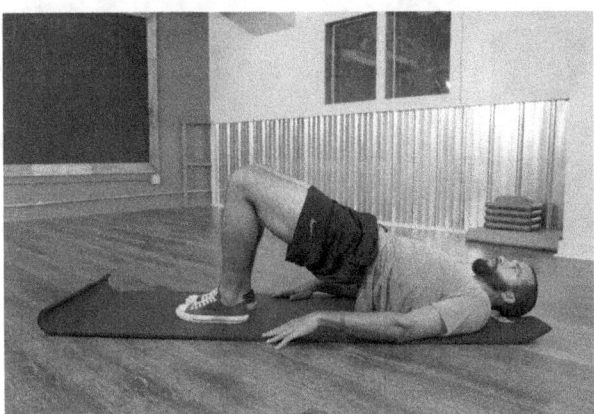

(b) Lift the butt off the floor.

Ideal ability: Able to perform a set of 20 repetitions with perfect form and minimal difficulty.

Perfect form includes: Able to achieve full hip extension. No loss of neutral spine/core engagement (the low back doesn't arch and/or ribs don't flair out). No hamstring cramping or low back tightness.

Not appropriate to perform if: Unable to lift butt off the ground, unable to maintain a neutral spine (back arches or ribs flair out), or movement causes pain.

If the double leg bridge exercise is appropriate to perform but form requires improvement, continue performing the double leg bridge exercise but work to improve form.

If the double leg bridge exercise is inappropriate to perform, work on engaging the core and gluts in the supine position with proper breathing.

BIRD DOG UE/LE PROGRESSION

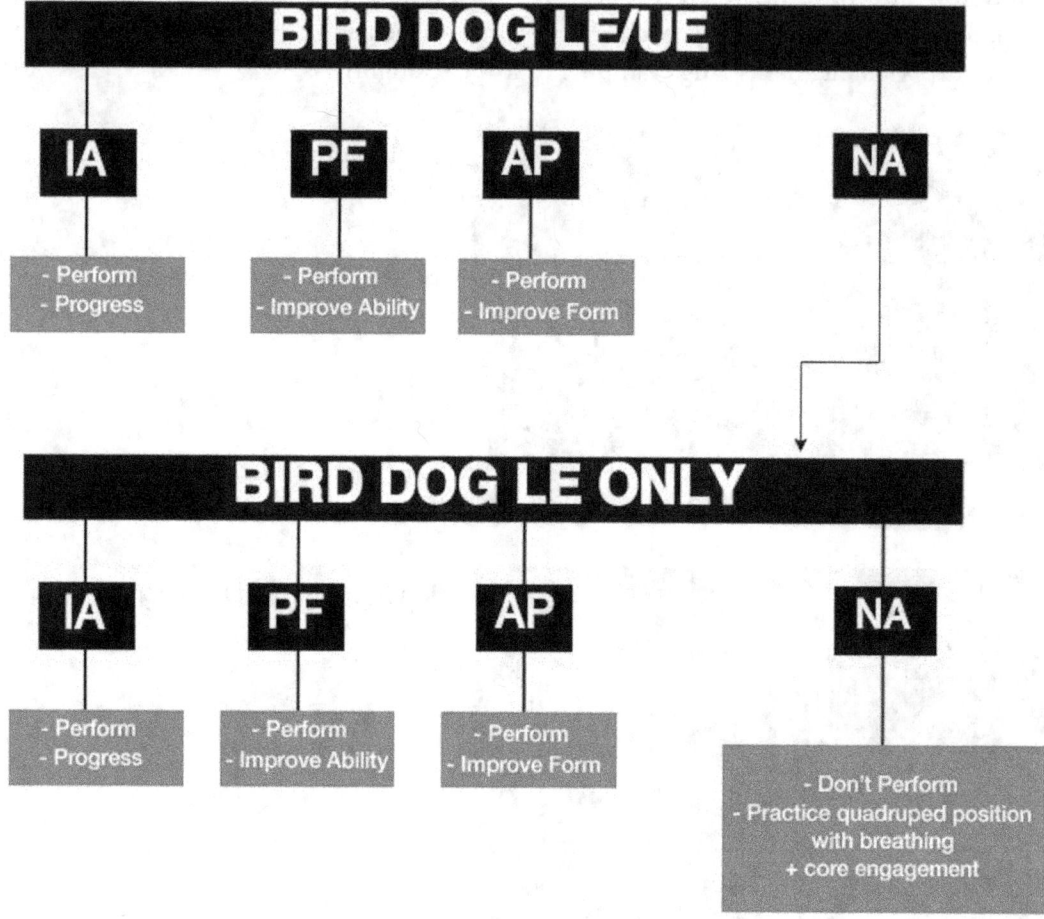

Positioning and Alignment

Prior to performing exercises in this position you must understand how to achieve proper alignment.

How to achieve proper quadruped positioning: Get on all fours with the hands under the shoulders and knees under the hips. Engage the core and perform diaphragmatic breathing.

Additional information: Maintain a neutral head and neck and low back position with the core engaged. Don't sag or round the back and avoid any shoulder shrugging. There should be a straight line from the head to the tail bone.

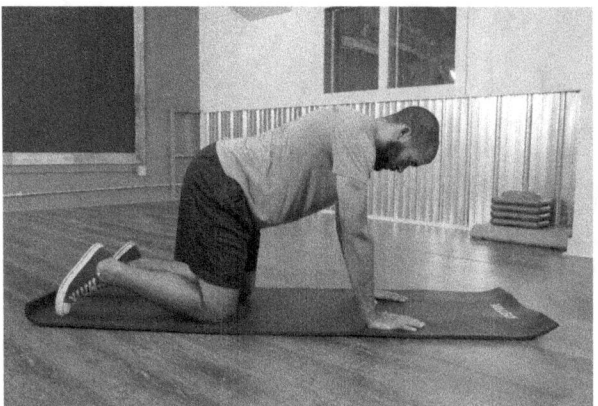

Proper Quadruped Positioning:
Hands under shoulders,
knees under hips;
neutral head and neck;
neutral low back;
core engaged

Things to look for:

— Are the hands under the shoulders and the knees under the hips?
— Is the head and neck neutral?
— Is the low back in a neutral position with the core engaged?
— Are the shoulders in a good position?
— Is the upper back overly rounded?
— Can you breathe properly without altering the position?

Bird Dog UE/LE

How to perform: Get on all fours with the knees under the hips and hands under the shoulders. Engage the core and extend one leg straight back while lifting the opposite arm out in front and pause. Bring the arm and leg back in, touching elbow to knee and extend back out.

Additional information: Maintain a neutral spine position without arching or rounding the low back, and keep the pelvis level throughout.

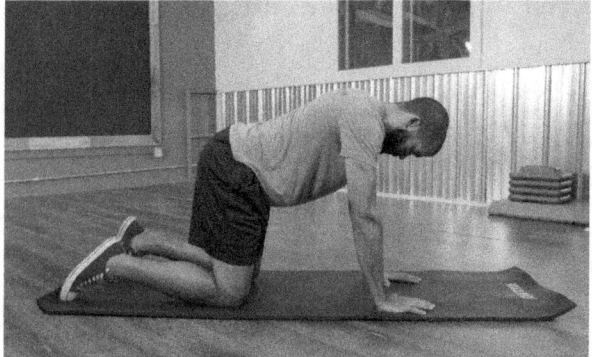

(a) Quadruped position;

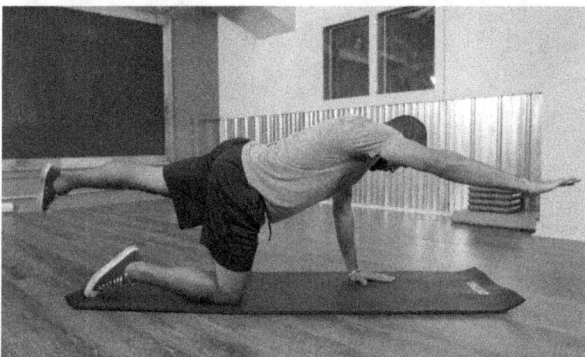

(b) Opposite arm and leg extended;

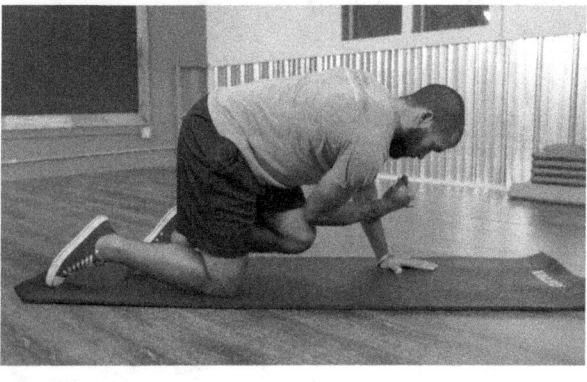

(c) Opposite knee to elbow.

Ideal ability: Able to perform a set of 10 repetitions on the right and left with perfect form and minimal difficulty.

Perfect form includes: Able to maintain balance and control with full extension and touching elbow to knee. No loss of neutral low back, head and neck, or shoulder positioning. Pelvis and trunk remain level throughout.

Inappropriate to perform if: Unable to complete movement due to complete loss of balance and control. Unable to maintain neutral low back, head and neck, or shoulder positioning, or if movement causes pain.

If the UE/LE bird dog exercise is appropriate to perform but form requires improvement, continue performing the UE/LE bird dog exercise while working to improve form.

If the UE/LE bird dog exercise is inappropriate to perform, assess if the LE-only bird dog exercise is appropriate to perform.

Bird Dog LE-Only

How to perform: Get on all fours with the knees under the hips and hands under the shoulders. Engage the core and extend one leg straight back and pause, then bring the leg back to the starting position.

Additional information: Maintain a neutral spine position without arching or rounding the low back, and keep the pelvis level throughout.

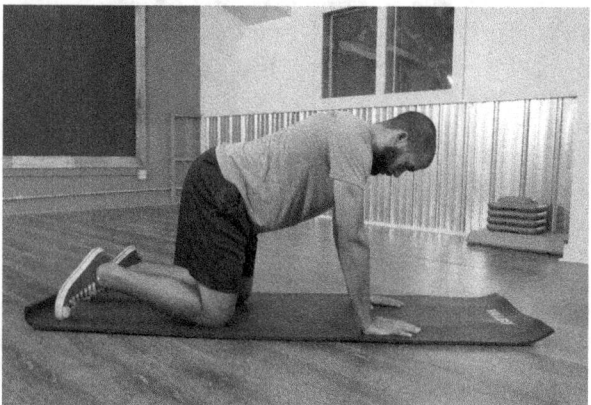

(a) Quadruped position;

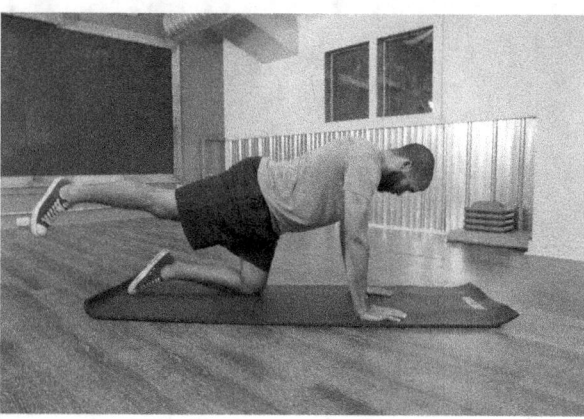

(b) Leg extended.

Ideal ability: Able to perform a set of 20 repetitions with perfect form and minimal difficulty.

Perfect form includes: Able to maintain balance and control with full leg extension. No loss of neutral low back, head and neck, or shoulder positioning. Pelvis and trunk remain level throughout.

Inappropriate to perform if: Unable to complete movement due to complete loss of balance and control. Unable to maintain neutral low back, head and neck, or shoulder positioning, or movement causes pain.

If the LE-only bird dog exercise is appropriate to perform but form requires improvement, continue performing the LE-only bird dog exercise while working to improve form.

If the LE-only bird dog exercise is inappropriate to perform, work on engaging the core and breathing while achieving proper positioning in the quadruped position.

PLANK PROGRESSION

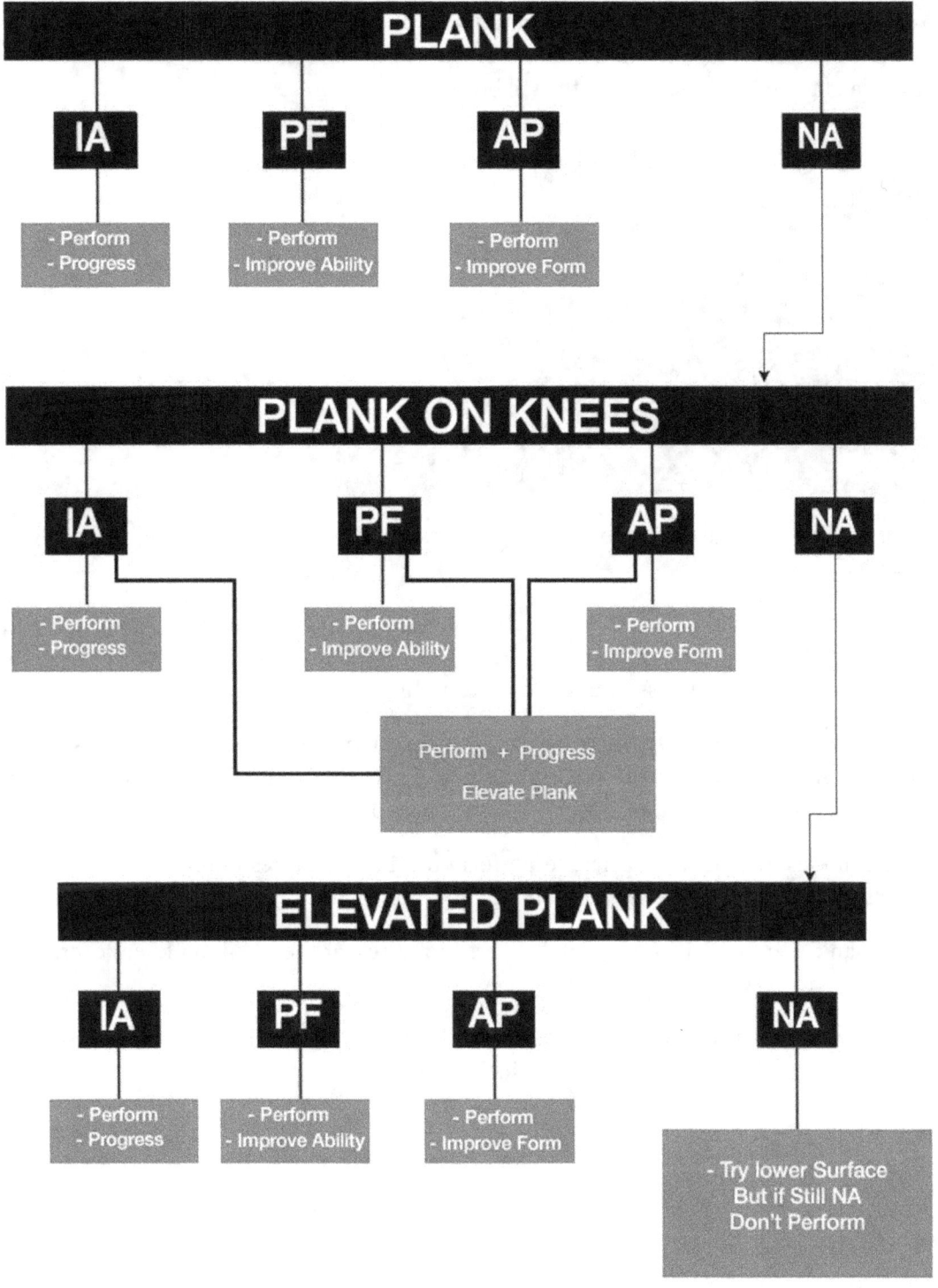

Plank

How to perform: Lie on your stomach and prop up on the forearms with the elbows under the shoulders. Lift up into a plank position and hold while engaging the core and squeezing the gluts.

Additional information: Maintain a neutral head and neck and low back position with the core engaged. Don't sag or round the back and avoid any shoulder shrugging. There should be a straight line from the head to the tail bone.

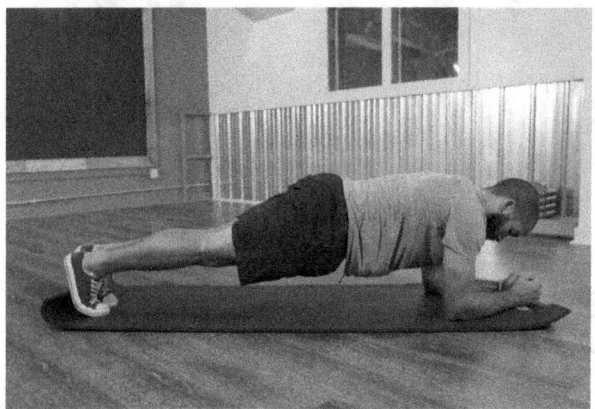

Elbows under shoulders;
neutral head and neck position;
neutral low back position;
core engaged.

Ideal ability: Able to hold the position for 60seconds with perfect form and minimal difficulty.

Perfect form includes: Elbows are directly under the shoulders. Neutral lumbar spine with core engaged. Neutral head and neck position. Good scapular and shoulder positioning (no shoulder shrugging or excessive upper back rounding).

Inappropriate to perform if: Unable to achieve or maintain neutral lumbar spine or unable to achieve and maintain neutral head and neck position. Unable to achieve good scapular and shoulder positioning or position causes pain.

If the plank exercise is appropriate to perform but form requires improvement, continue performing the plank exercise while working to improve form.

If the plank exercise is inappropriate to perform, assess if the plank on knees exercise is appropriate to perform.

How to progress the plank exercise or make harder: Perform the plank exercise with arms on an unstable surface. Perform a single leg plank.

Plank on Knees

How to perform: Lie on your stomach and prop up on the forearms with the elbows under the shoulders. Lift up into a plank position on the knees and hold while engaging the core and squeezing the gluts.

Additional information: Maintain a neutral head and neck and low back position with the core engaged. Don't sag or round the back and avoid any shoulder shrugging. There should be a straight line from the head to the tail bone.

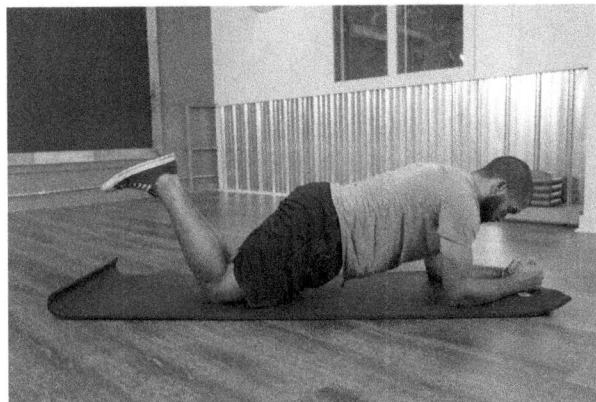

Plank position on knees.

Ideal ability: Able to hold the position for 60 seconds with perfect form and minimal difficulty.

Perfect form includes: Elbows are directly under the shoulders. Neutral lumbar spine with core engaged. Neutral head and neck position with postural muscles engaged. Good scapular and shoulder positioning (no shoulder shrugging or excessive upper back rounding).

Inappropriate to perform if: Unable to achieve or maintain neutral lumbar spine. Unable to achieve and maintain neutral head and neck position. Unable to achieve good scapular and shoulder positioning or position causes pain.

If the plank on knees exercise is appropriate to perform but the form requires improvement, continue performing the plank on knees exercise while working to improve form. Perform the elevated plank exercise and progress by lowering the surface until able to perform the plank with elbows on the ground.

If the plank on knees exercise is inappropriate to perform, assess if the elevated plank exercise is appropriate to perform (assess using any surface height).

Elevated Plank

How to perform: Rest the forearms on an elevated surface. Lift up into a plank position and hold while engaging the core and squeezing the gluts.

Additional information: Maintain a neutral head and neck and low back position with the core engaged. Don't sag or round the back and avoid any shoulder shrugging. There should be a straight line from the head to the tail bone.

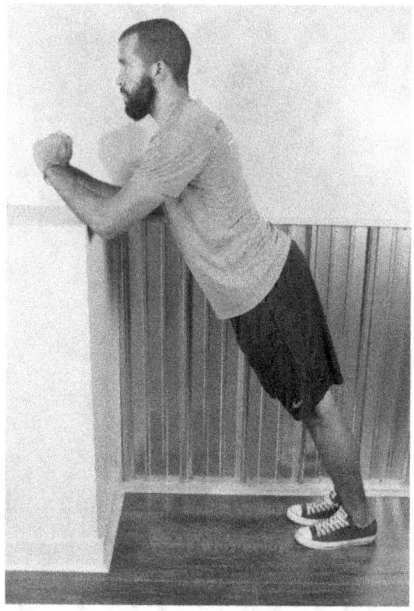

Elevated plank position

Ideal ability: Able to hold the position (at any given surface height) for at least 60 seconds with perfect form and minimal difficulty.

Perfect form includes: Elbows are directly under the shoulders, neutral lumbar spine with core engaged. Neutral head and neck position with postural muscles engaged. Good scapular and shoulder positioning (no shoulder shrugging or excessive upper back rounding).

Inappropriate to perform if: Unable to achieve or maintain neutral lumbar spine. Unable to achieve and maintain neutral head and neck position. Unable to achieve good scapular and shoulder positioning or if position causes pain.

If the elevated plank exercise is appropriate to perform but the form requires improvement, continue performing the elevated plank exercise while working to improve form. Slowly progress by using a lower support surface.

If the elevated plank exercise is inappropriate to perform, first try using a higher surface to make the exercise easier but, if still inappropriate, hold off on performing planks.

How to progress or make harder: Lower the support surface.

SIDE PLANK PROGRESSION

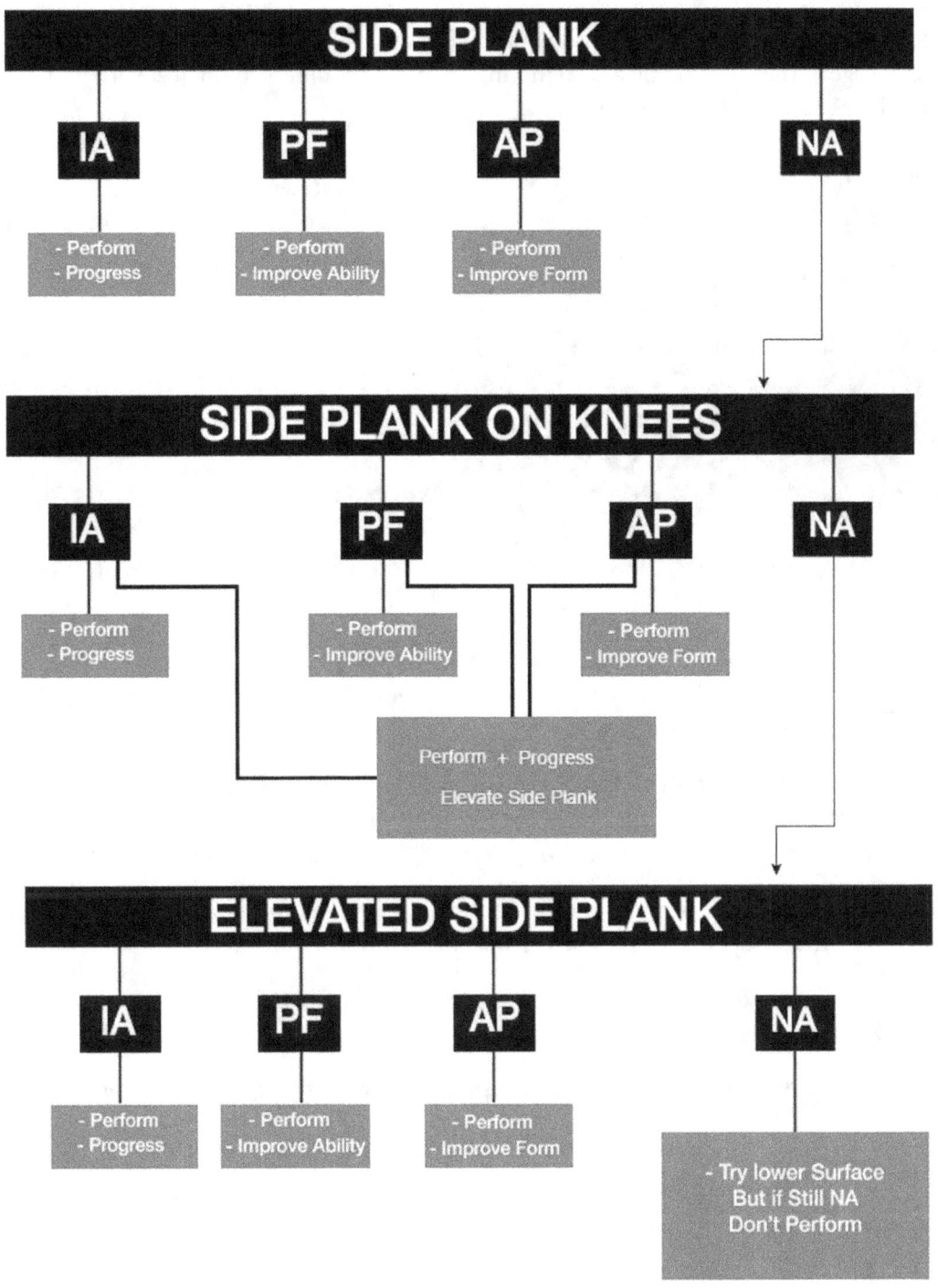

Side Plank

How to perform: Lie on your side propped up on the forearm with the elbow under the shoulder. Lift up into a side plank position and hold while engaging the core and squeezing the gluts.

Additional information: Maintain a neutral head and neck and low back position with the core engaged. There should be a straight line from the shoulders to the feet with no flexion in the hips or rotation of the trunk.

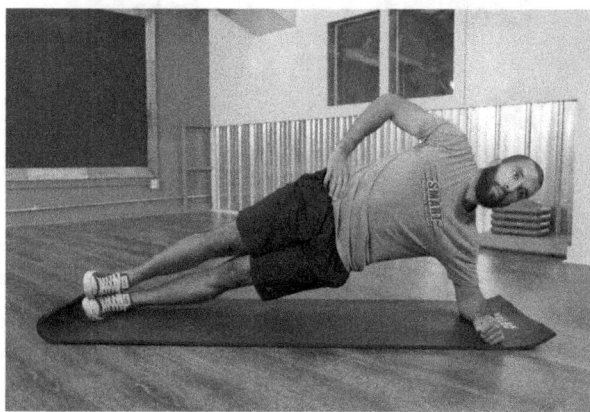

Elbow under shoulder;
Shoulder, hips, and feet aligned;
neutral low back position;
core engaged.

Ideal ability: Able to hold the position for 30 seconds with perfect form and minimal difficulty.

Perfect form includes: The elbow is directly under the shoulder. The body is in a straight line with no flexion of the hips or rotation of the shoulders and trunk. The head and neck and low back are in a neutral position.

Inappropriate to perform if: Unable to balance and support the body in the position or unable to achieve a straight line with no flexion of the hips or trunk rotation. Unable to achieve a neutral head and neck and low back position, or if position causes pain.

If the side plank exercise is appropriate to perform but form requires improvement, continue performing the side plank exercise while working to improve form.

If the side plank exercise is inappropriate to perform, assess if the side plank on knees exercise is appropriate to perform.

How to progress the side plank exercise or make harder: Perform a single leg side plank.

Side Plank on Knees

How to perform: Lie on your side and prop up on the forearm with the elbow under the shoulder. Lift up into a side plank position on the knees and hold while engaging the core and squeezing the gluts.

Additional information: Maintain a neutral head and neck and low back position with the core engaged. There should be a straight line from the shoulders to the knees with no flexion in the hips or rotation of the trunk.

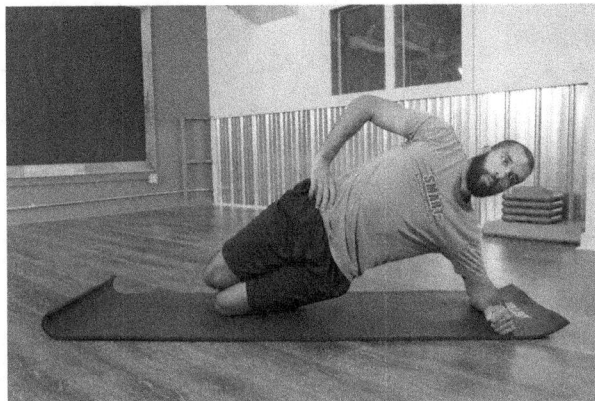

Side plank position on knees.

Ideal ability: Able to hold the position for 30 seconds with perfect form and minimal difficulty.

Perfect form includes: The elbow is directly under the shoulder. The body is in a straight line with no flexion of the hips or rotation of the shoulders and trunk. The head and neck and low back are in a neutral position.

Inappropriate to perform if: Unable to balance and support the body in the position or unable to achieve a straight line with no flexion of the hips or trunk rotation. Unable to achieve a neutral head and neck and low back position, or if position causes pain.

If the side plank on knees exercise is appropriate to perform but form requires improvement, continue performing the side plank on knees exercise and working to improve form. Perform the elevated side plank exercise and lower the surface height until able to perform side plank with the elbow on the floor.

If the side plank on knees exercise is inappropriate to perform, assess if the elevated side plank exercise is appropriate to perform (assess using any support height).

Elevated Side Plank

How to perform: Face sideways and rest one forearm on an elevated surface. Lift up into a side plank position and hold while engaging the core and squeezing the gluts.

Additional Information: Maintain a neutral head and neck and low back position with the core engaged. There should be a straight line from the shoulders to the feet with no flexion in the hips or rotation of the trunk.

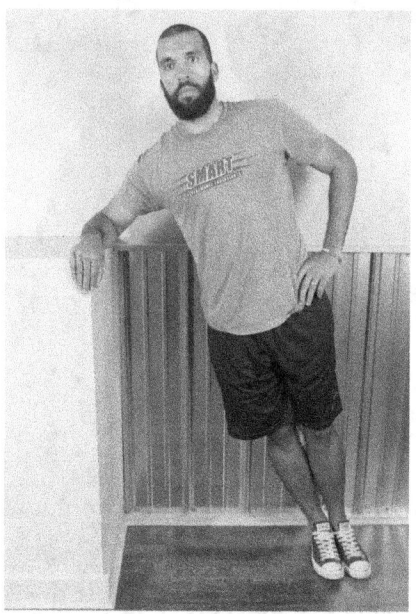

Elevated side plank position.

Ideal ability: Able to hold the position for 30 seconds (at a given surface height) with perfect form and minimal difficulty.

Perfect form includes: The elbow is directly under the shoulder. The body is in a straight line with no flexion of the hips or rotation of the shoulders and trunk. The head and neck and low back are in a neutral position.

Inappropriate to perform if: Unable to balance and support the body in the position or unable to achieve a straight line with no flexion of the hips or trunk rotation. Unable to achieve a neutral head and neck and low back position or if position causes pain.

If the elevated side plank exercise is appropriate to perform but form requires improvement, continue performing the elevated side plank exercise while working to improve form and slowly progress by lowering the support surface.

If the elevated side plank exercise is inappropriate to perform, first try using a higher surface to make the exercise easier but, if still inappropriate, hold off on performing any side plank exercise.

How to progress or make harder: Perform on a lower surface.

PUSH UP PROGRESSION

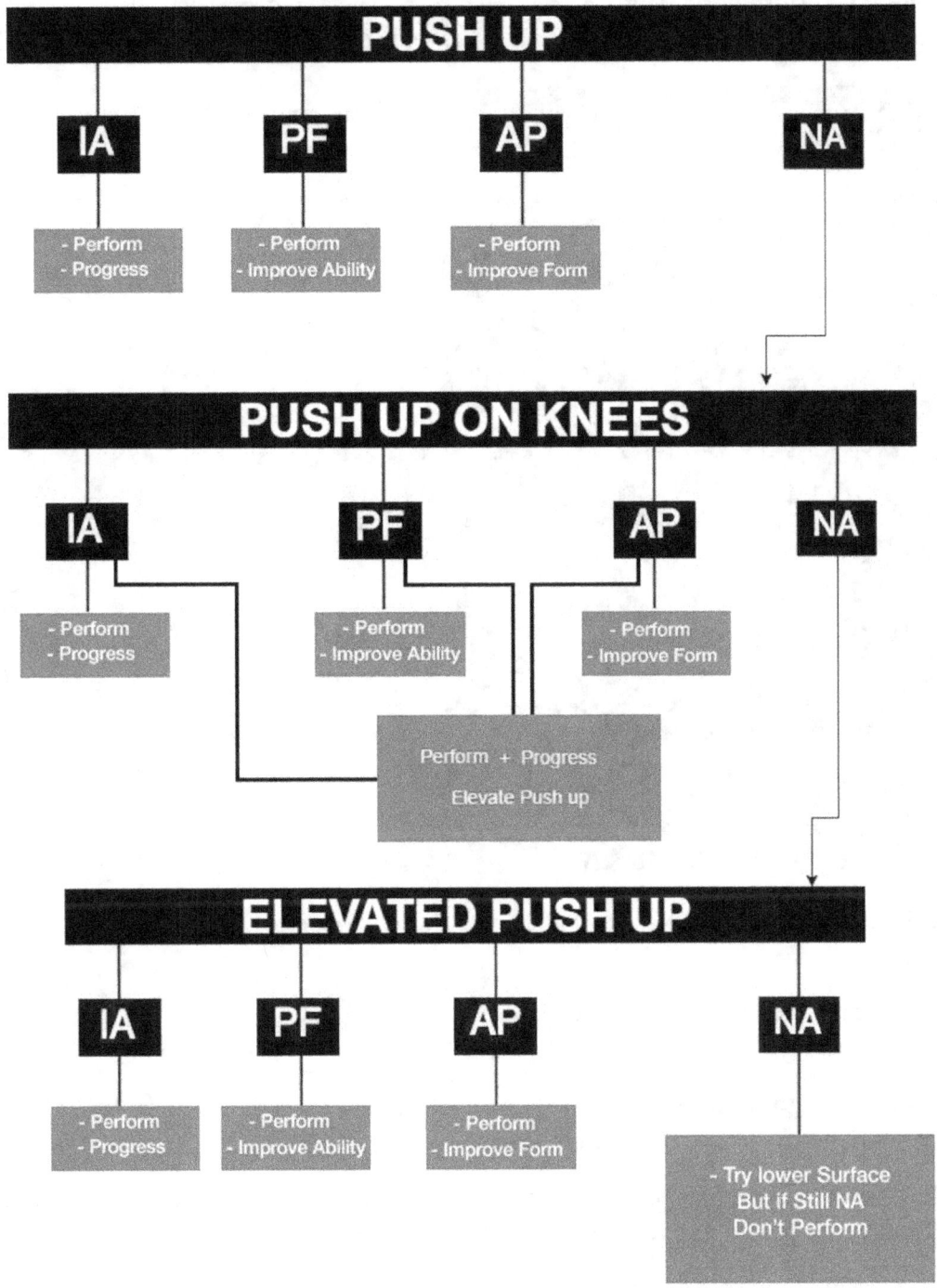

Push Up

How to perform: Get into a push up position. Engage the core and squeeze the gluts, then lower the body letting the elbows bend to 90 degrees and push back up.

Additional information: Maintain a neutral head and neck and low back position with the core engaged. Don't sag or round the back and avoid any shoulder shrugging.

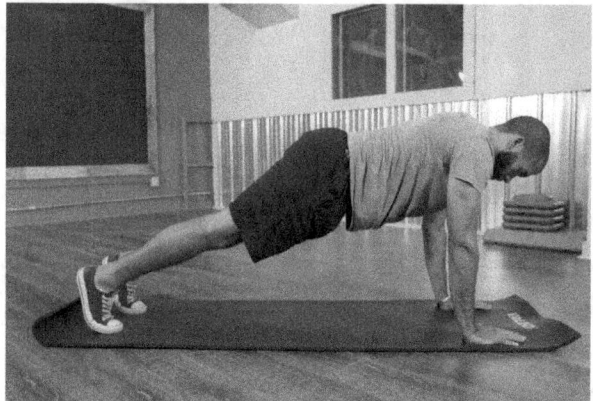

(a) Push up position;

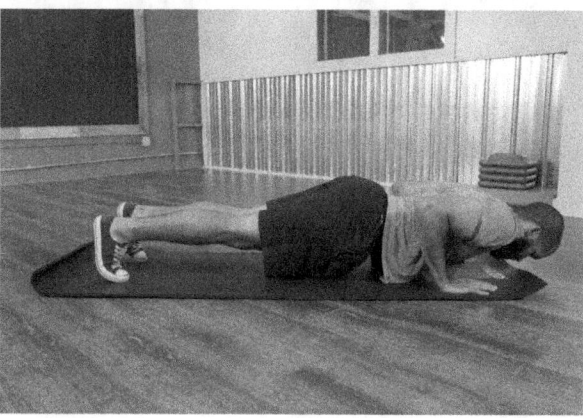

(b) Lower body into the push up.

Ideal ability: Able to complete a set of 20 repetitions with perfect form and minimal difficulty.

Perfect form includes: Able to lower the body, bending the elbows to at least 90 degrees and push back up. No loss of head and neck, shoulder, or low back positioning.

Inappropriate to perform if: Unable to maintain good head and neck, shoulder, and low back position throughout, or if the movement causes pain.

If the push up exercise is appropriate to perform but form requires improvement, continue performing the push up exercise while working to improve form.

If the push up exercise is inappropriate to perform, assess if the push up on knees exercise is appropriate to perform.

Push Up on Knees

How to perform: Get into a push up position on the knees. Engage the core and squeeze the gluts, then lower the body, letting the elbows bend to 90 degrees and push back up.

Additional information: Maintain a neutral head and neck and low back position with the core engaged. Don't sag or round the back and avoid any shoulder shrugging.

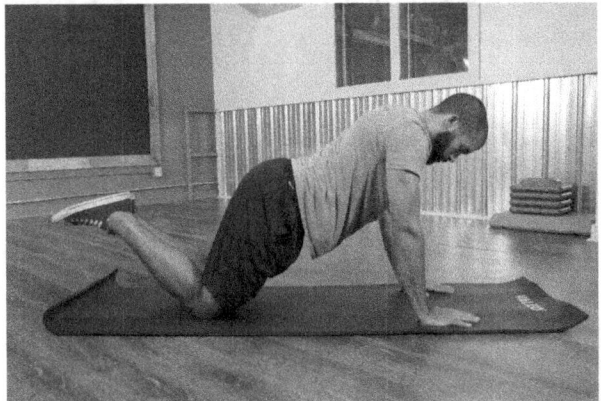

(a) Push up position on knees;

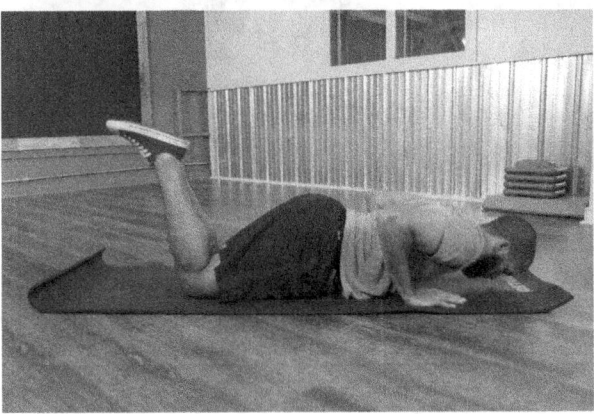

(b) Lower body into push up.

Ideal ability: Able to perform a set of 20 repetitions with perfect form and minimal difficulty.

Perfect form includes: Able to lower the body, bending the elbows to at least 90 degrees and push back up. No loss of head and neck, shoulder, and low back positioning.

Inappropriate to perform if: Unable to maintain good head and neck, shoulder, and low back position throughout, or if the movement causes pain

If the push up on knees exercise is appropriate to perform but form requires improvement, continue performing the push up on knees exercise while working to improve form. Perform the elevated push up exercise and progress by lowering the surface until able to do a push up with the hands on the floor.

If the push up on knees exercise is inappropriate, assess if the elevated push up exercise is appropriate to perform (assess using any surface height).

Elevated Push Up

How to perform: Get into a push up position with the hands on an elevated surface. Engage the core and squeeze the gluts, then lower the body, letting the elbows bend to 90 degrees and push back up.

Additional information: Maintain a neutral head and neck and low back position with the core engaged. Don't sag or round the back and avoid any shoulder shrugging.

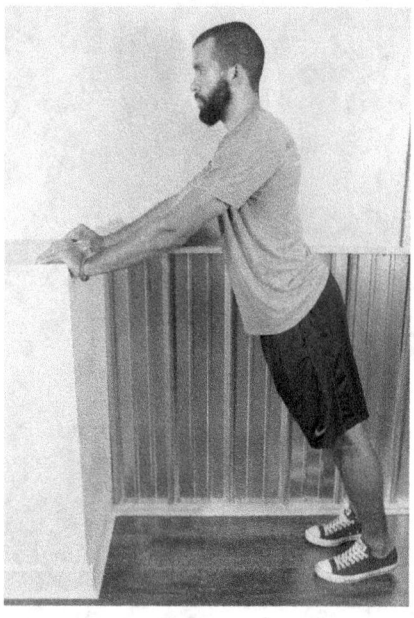 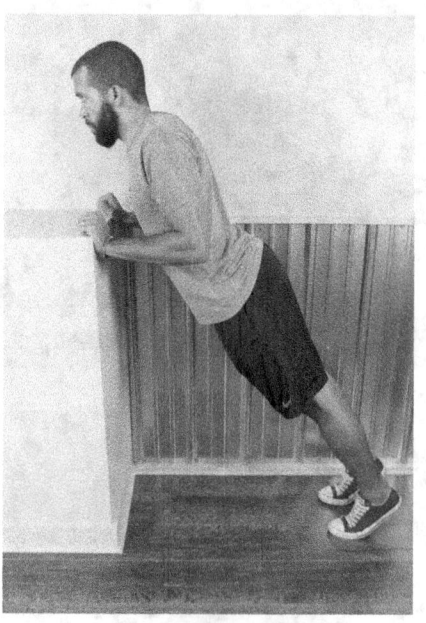

(a) Elevated push up position;   (b) Lower body into push up.

Ideal ability: Able to perform a set of 20 repetitions (at a given surface height) with perfect form and minimal difficulty.

Perfect form includes: Able to lower the body, bending the elbows to at least 90 degrees and push back up. No loss of head and neck, shoulder, and low back positioning.

Inappropriate to perform if: Unable to maintain good head and neck, shoulder, and low back position throughout, or if the movement causes pain.

If the elevated push up exercise is appropriate to perform but the form requires improvement, continue performing the elevated push up exercise while working to improve form. Slowly progress by lowering the support surface.

If the elevated push up exercise is inappropriate to perform, first try elevating the surface (up to a wall push up if necessary) but if still inappropriate, hold off on doing pushups.

How to progress or make harder: Lower the surface height.

RDL PROGRESSION (Double Leg)

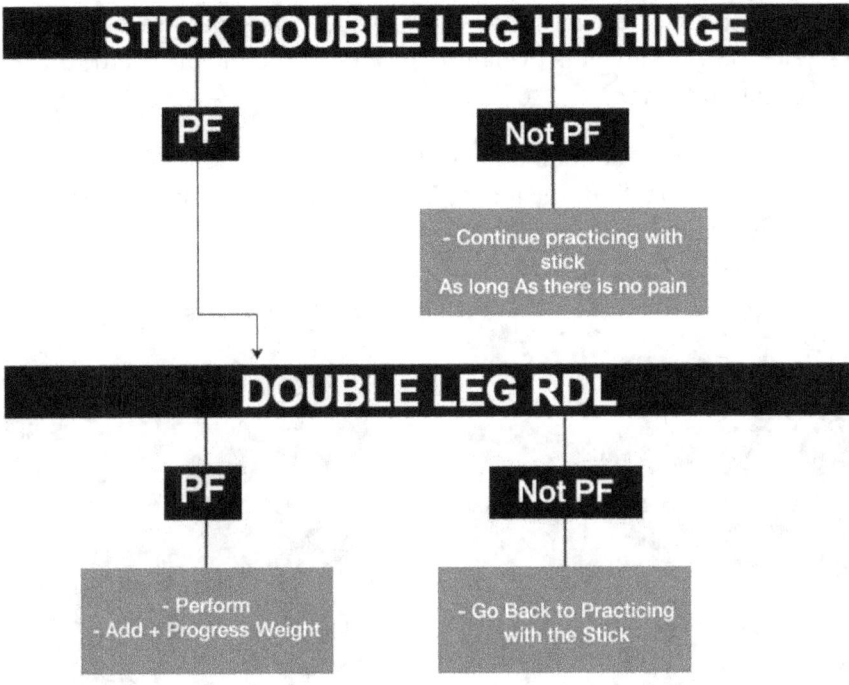

STICK DOUBLE LEG HIP HINGE

PF

Not PF
- Continue practicing with stick
As long As there is no pain

DOUBLE LEG RDL

PF
- Perform
- Add + Progress Weight

Not PF
- Go Back to Practicing with the Stick

RDL PROGRESSION (Single Leg)

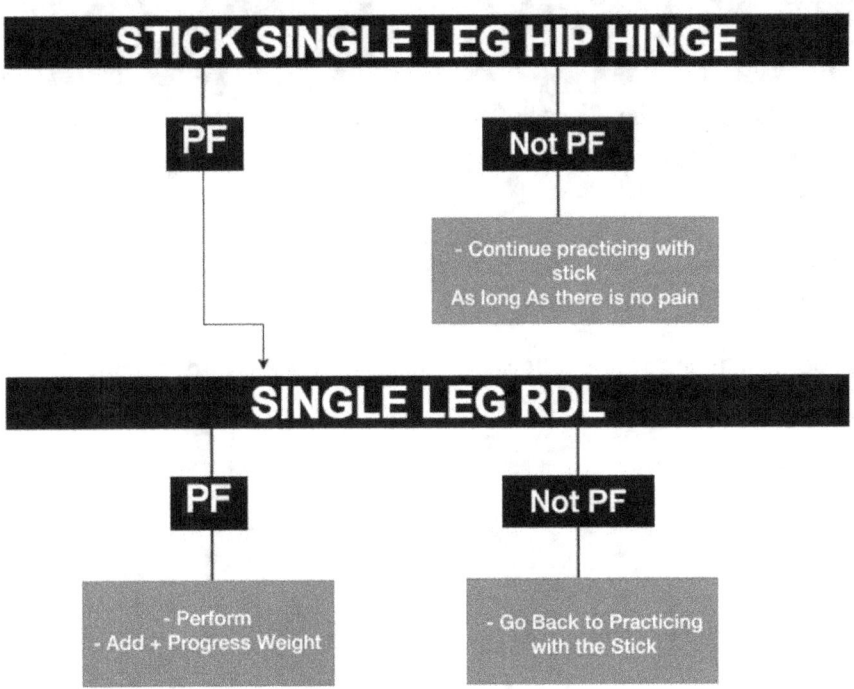

STICK SINGLE LEG HIP HINGE

PF

Not PF
- Continue practicing with stick
As long As there is no pain

SINGLE LEG RDL

PF
- Perform
- Add + Progress Weight

Not PF
- Go Back to Practicing with the Stick

Stick Double Leg Hip Hinge

How to perform: Stand with feet shoulder-width apart and toes facing forward. Hold a stick behind the back with one hand in the small of the back and the other behind the neck. Engage the core and squeeze the gluts, then sit the butt back and hinge forward at the hips until you feel tension in the gluts or hamstrings. Push the hips forward to come back up squeezing the gluts at the top.

Additional information: Maintain a neutral spine and keep the stick in contact with the head, back, and butt throughout the movement. Keep the knees in a relaxed stance without flexing or hyperextending.

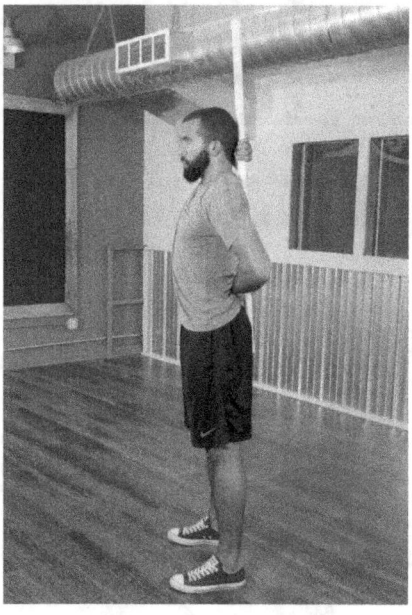
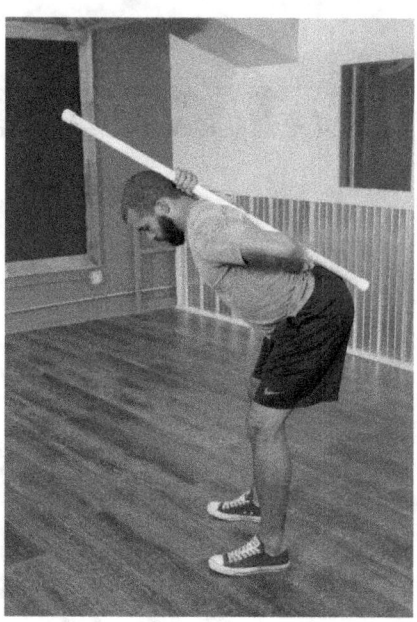

(a) Stand with feet shoulder-width apart, toes facing forward holding a stick behind the back;

(b) Hinge forward at the hips

Proper form requires: No spinal flexion—the stick remains in contact with the head, back, and butt. No flexion or hyperextension of the knees. The hips and butt shift backward.

If form is good and the movement does not cause pain, assess if the double leg RDL exercise is appropriate to perform.

Double Leg RDL

How to perform: Stand with feet shoulder-width apart and toes facing forward. Engage the core and squeeze the gluts, then sit the butt back and hinge forward at the hips until you feel tension in the gluts or hamstrings. Push the hips forward to come back up, squeezing the gluts at the top.

Additional information: Maintain a neutral head and neck and low back throughout the movement. Keep the knees in a relaxed stance without flexing or hyperextending.

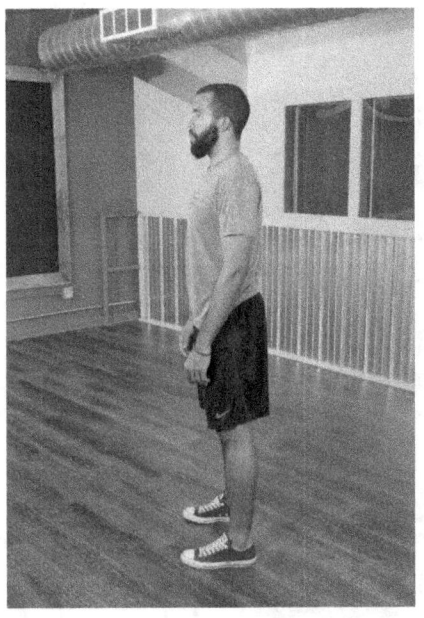 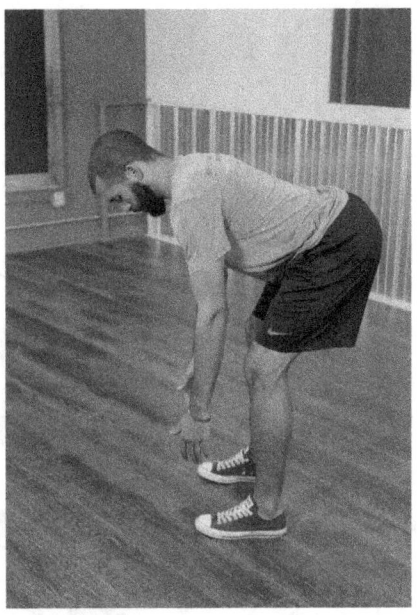

(a) Stand feet shoulder-width apart, toes facing forward;

(b) Hinge forward at the hips.

Ideal ability: Able to complete a set of 10 repetitions with perfect form and minimal difficulty using a 20 lb. weight.

Perfect form includes: The head and neck, shoulders, and low back remain in a neutral position throughout. The hips and butt move backward as the trunk flexes forward without bending in the spine. The knees maintain a soft knee stance without flexing or hyperextension.

If form is not perfect, go back to practicing the stick double leg hip hinge exercise.

If form is perfect, add weight.

How to progress or make harder: Add more weight.

Single Leg Balance

Prior to learning the single leg hip hinge, screen for adequate single leg balance. If balance is not adequate, hold off on learning the single leg hip hinge until single leg balance improves.

Adequate single leg balance: Able to stand on right and left leg for at least 10 seconds with no trunk movement and arms at the side.

Ideal single leg balance: Able to stand on right and left leg for at least 30 seconds with no trunk movement and arms at the side.

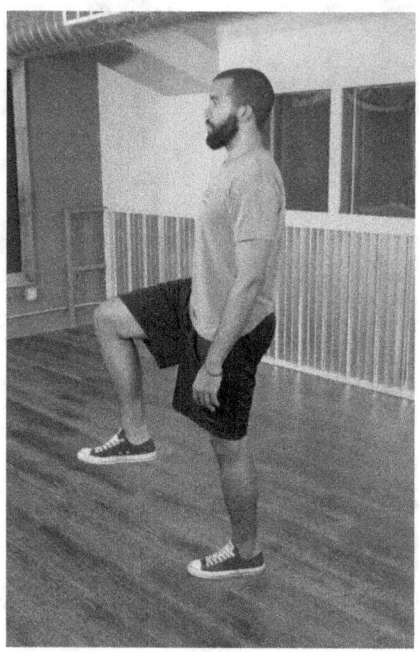

Stand and balance on one leg.

To address inadequate single leg balance: Stand in a doorway and lift one knee up to 90 degrees while lightly pushing back against the wall with the hands. Once you feel stable, slowly lift the hands off the wall and try to balance. If you lose balance, use the wall to steady yourself.

Assisted Single Leg Balance

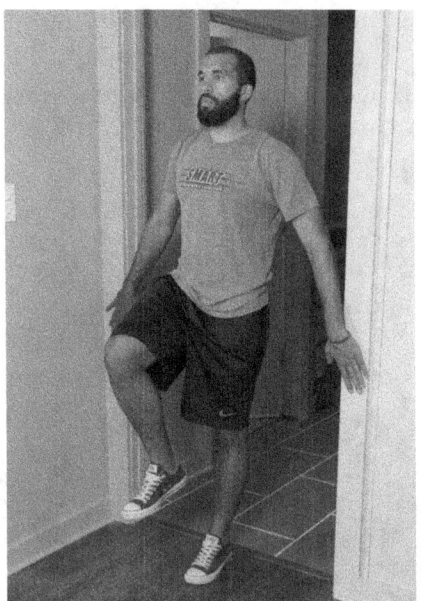 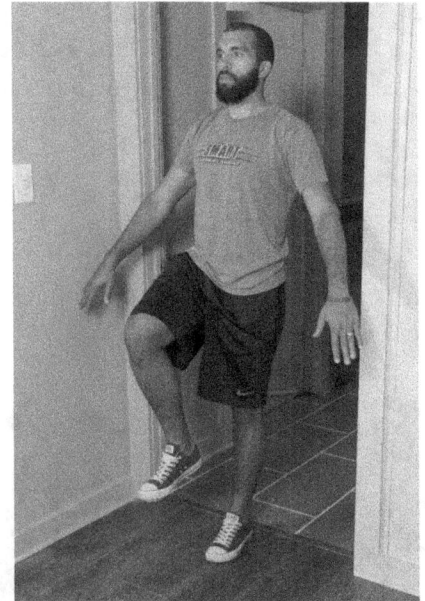

(a) Balance on one leg with hands pushing on doorway to help balance;

(b) Lift hand off doorway and continue balancing.

Stick Single Leg Hip Hinge

How to perform: Stand feet together toes facing forward. Hold a stick behind the back with one hand in the small of the back and the other behind the neck. Engage the core and squeeze the gluts, then sit the butt back and hinge forward at the hip on one leg until you feel tension in the stance glut and hamstring. Push the hip forward to come back up, squeezing the gluts at the top.

Additional information: Maintain a neutral spine and keep the stick in contact with the head, back, and butt throughout the movement. Keep the stance knee in a relaxed stance without flexing or hyperextending. Also, keep the back leg in line with the body as you hinge forward.

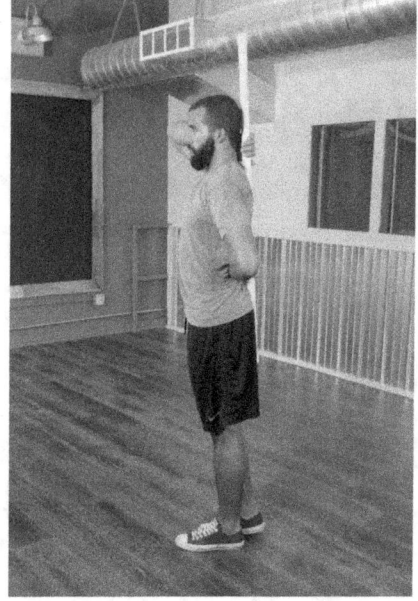 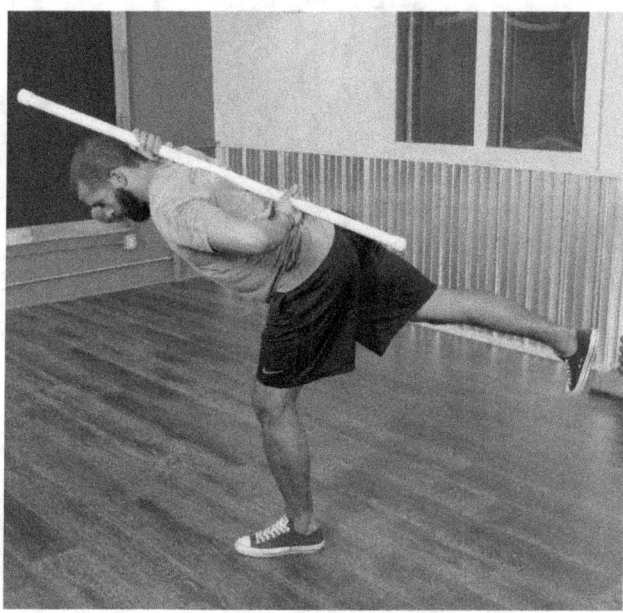

(a) Stand feet together, toes facing forward holding a stick behind the back;

(b) Hinge forward at the hips on one leg.

Proper form requirements: The stick remains in contact with the head, back, and butt. No flexion or hyperextension of the knees. The hips and butt shift backward. The non-stance leg remains in line with the trunk.

If form is good and the movement does not cause pain, assess if the single leg RDL exercise is appropriate to perform.

Single Leg RDL

How to perform: Stand feet together and toes facing forward. Engage the core and squeeze the gluts, then sit the butt back and hinge forward, bending at the hip on one leg until you feel tension in the stance glut or hamstring. Push the hip forward to come back up squeezing the gluts at the top.

Additional information: Maintain a neutral head and neck and low back throughout the movement. Keep the stance knee in a relaxed stance without flexing or hyperextending. Also, keep the back leg in line with the trunk as you hinge forward.

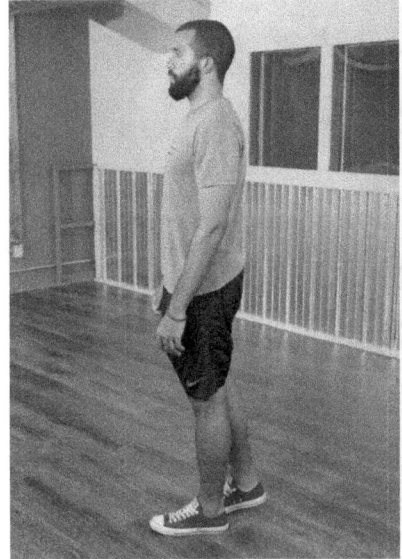 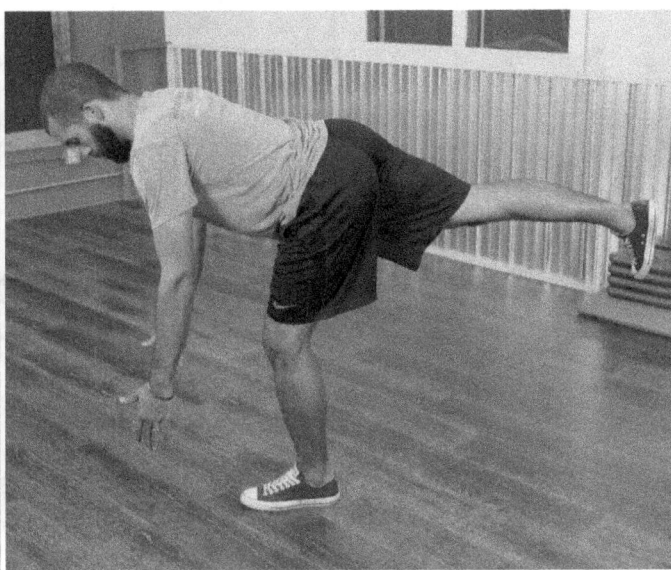

(a) Stand feet together, toes facing forward;

(b) Hinge forward at the hips on one leg.

Ideal ability: Able to complete a set of 10 repetitions on the right and left with perfect form and minimal difficulty using a 10 lb. weight.

Perfect form includes: The head and neck, shoulders, and low back remain in a neutral position throughout. The hips and butt move backward as the trunk flexes forward without bending in the spine. The stance knees maintain a soft knee bend stance without flexing or hyperextension. The back leg remains in line with the trunk.

If form is not perfect, go back to practicing the stick single leg hip hinge exercise.

If form is perfect, add weight.

How to progress or make harder: Add more weight.

STEP BACK LUNGE PROGRESSION

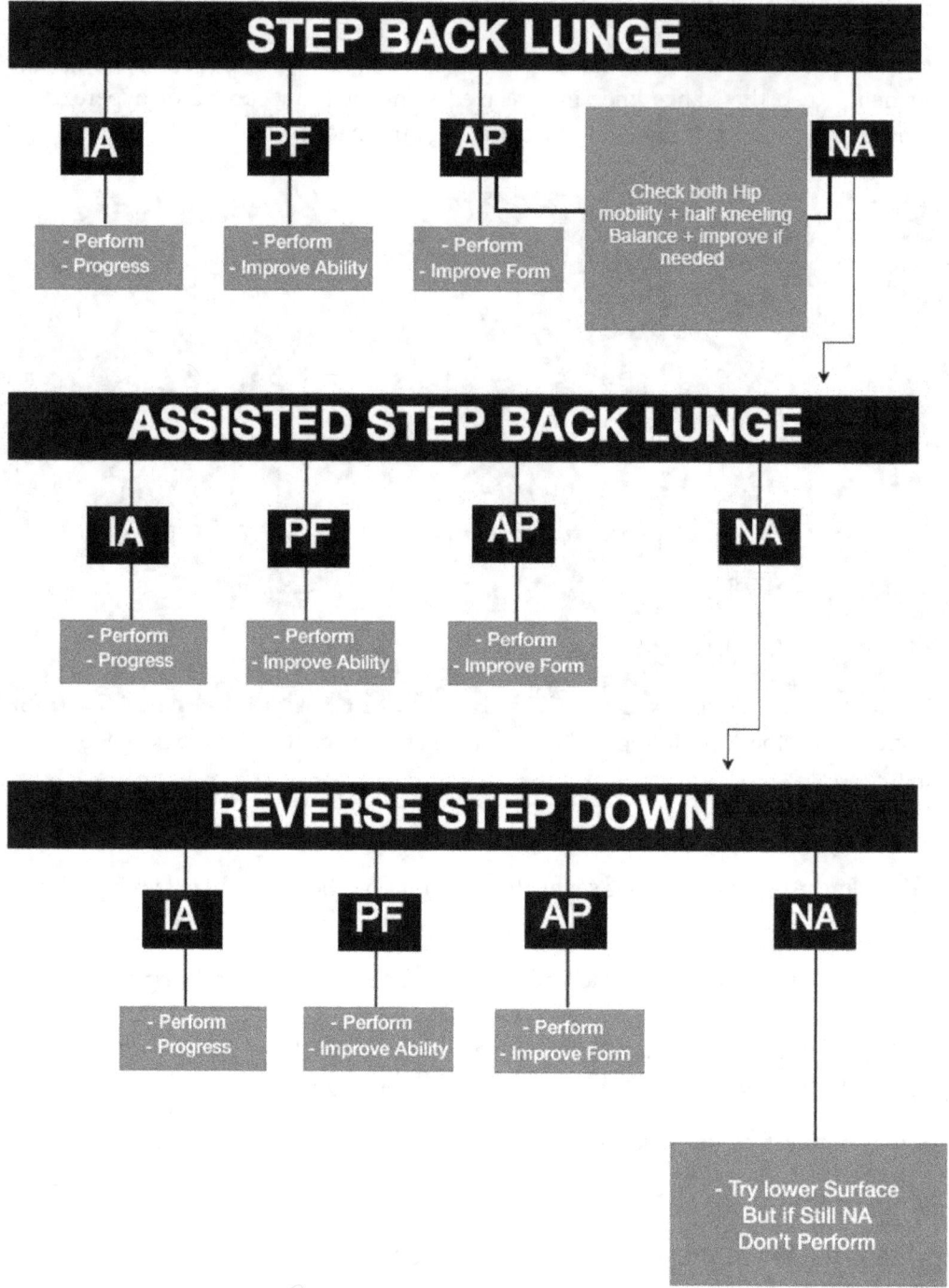

STEP BACK LUNGE

IA
- Perform
- Progress

PF
- Perform
- Improve Ability

AP
- Perform
- Improve Form

Check both Hip mobility + half kneeling Balance + improve if needed

NA

ASSISTED STEP BACK LUNGE

IA
- Perform
- Progress

PF
- Perform
- Improve Ability

AP
- Perform
- Improve Form

NA

REVERSE STEP DOWN

IA
- Perform
- Progress

PF
- Perform
- Improve Ability

AP
- Perform
- Improve Form

NA

- Try lower Surface
But if Still NA
Don't Perform

Step Back Lunge

How to perform: Stand with feet together and toes facing forward. Step straight back into a lunge with the front and back foot in line and stand back up.

Additional information: In a proper lunge position, the trunk remains upright, the front knee remains vertical, and back hip is fully extended and aligned with the knee.

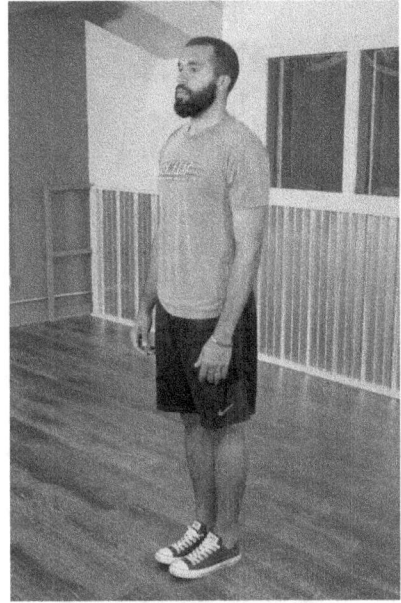
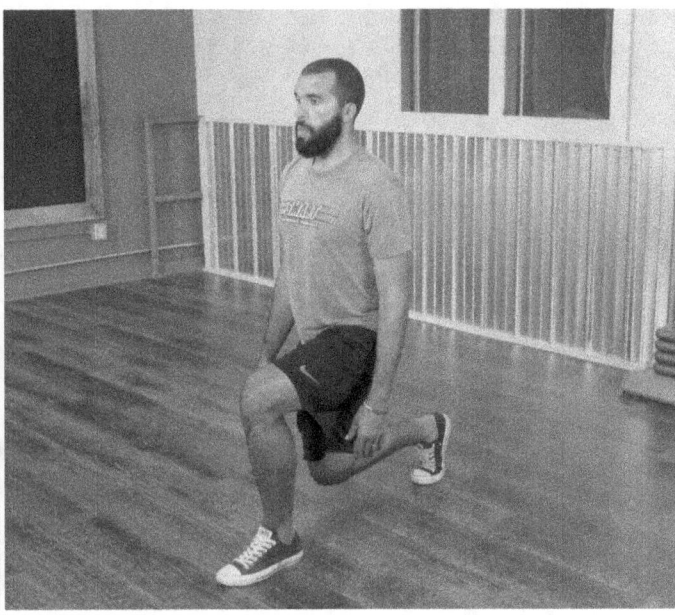

(a) Stand with feet together, toes facing forward;

(b) Step back into a lunge position.

Ideal ability: Able to complete a set of 20 repetitions on the right and left with perfect form and minimal difficulty.

Perfect form includes: Able to achieve lunge position with the feet in line and stand back up. Able to maintain balance and an upright trunk. The back hip and knee are aligned at the bottom of the lunge (butt doesn't sit back). The front knee doesn't collapse in or move forward.

Inappropriate to perform if: Unable to maintain balance and control during the movement. Unable to maintain a vertical tibia (knee collapses in or goes past the toes). Unable to keep the back hip and knee in alignment, or movement causes pain.

If the step back lunge exercise is appropriate to perform but form requires improvement, continue performing the step back lunge exercise while working to improve form. Check half-kneeling stance and work to improve it if limited (see Half-kneeling Balance on page 53). Check hip flexor mobility and work to improve it if limited (see *Mobility and Stretching* section for how to assess and improve hip flexor mobility).

If the step back lunge exercise is inappropriate to perform, assess if the assisted step back lunge exercise is appropriate to perform. Check half-kneeling stance and work to improve it if limited (see Half-kneeling Balance on page 53). Check hip flexor mobility and work to improve it if limited (see *Mobility and Stretching* section for how to assess and improve hip flexor mobility).

How to progress the step back lunge exercise or make harder: Add weight.

Assisted Step Back Lunge

How to perform: Stand with feet together and toes facing forward with one hand resting on a wall or stable object for balance. Step back into a lunge with the feet in line and stand back up using the hand for support.

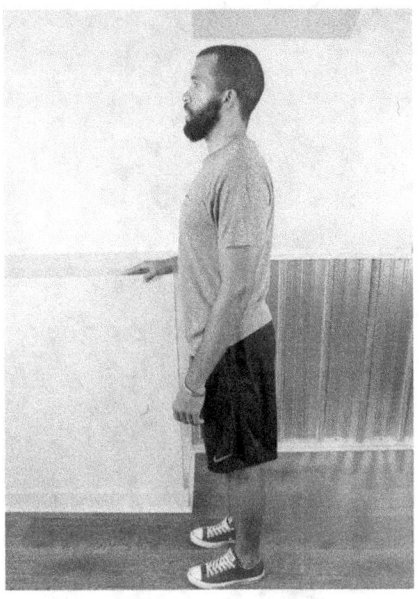

(a) Stand with feet together, toes facing forward, with your hand on a sturdy object;

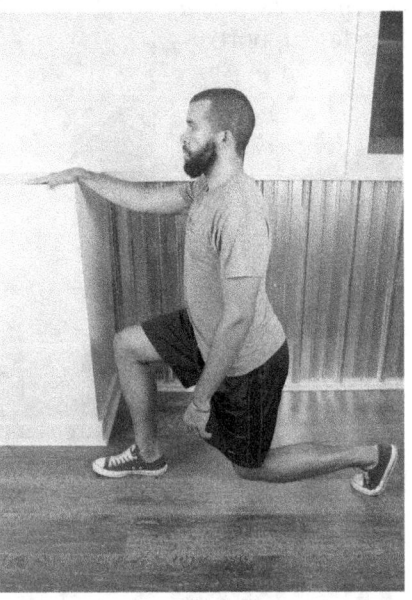

(b) Step back into lunge position.

Additional information: In a proper lunge position the trunk remains upright, the front knee remains vertical, and back hip is fully extended and aligned with the knee.

Ideal ability: Able to complete a set of 20 repetitions on the right and left with perfect form and minimal difficulty.

Perfect form includes: Able to achieve the lunge position with the feet in line and stand back up. Able to maintain an upright trunk. The back hip and knee are aligned at the bottom of the lunge (butt doesn't sit back). The knee doesn't collapse in or go forward.

Inappropriate to perform if: Unable to maintain control during the movement. Unable to maintain a vertical tibia (knee collapses in or goes past the toes). Unable to keep the back hip and knee in alignment, or movement causes pain.

If the assisted step back lunge exercise is appropriate to perform but form requires improvement, continue performing the assisted step back lunge exercise while working to improve form.

If the assisted step back lunge exercise is inappropriate to perform, assess if the reverse step down exercise is appropriate to perform.

Reverse Step Down

How to perform: Stand with feet together and toes facing forward on a step. In a slow and controlled movement, step down backwards off the step with one foot and come back up.

Additional information: Maintain an upright trunk. Keep the knee in a vertical position without going forward or collapsing inward. If you have difficulty balancing, hold on to something for support.

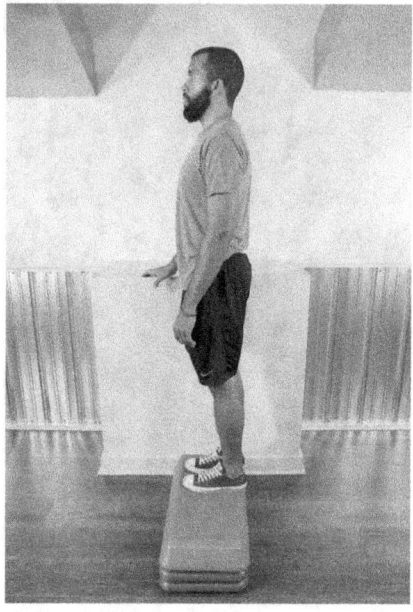 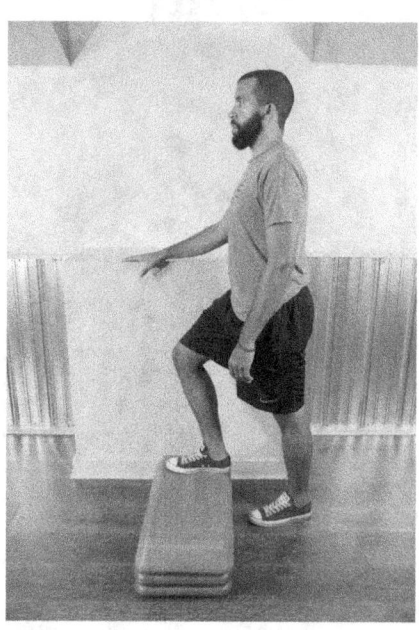

(a) Stand with feet together;   (b) Step down in a slow and
                                     controlled movement.

Ideal ability: Able to complete a set of 20 repetitions on the right and left with perfect form and minimal difficulty using a 10-inch step height.

Perfect form includes: Demonstrate control during the step down and back up. Trunk remains upright. Front knee doesn't collapse in or go forward (vertical tibia).

Inappropriate to perform if: Unable to prevent the knee from collapsing in or going forward past the toes, or if movement causes pain.

If the reverse step down exercise is appropriate to perform but form requires improvement, continue performing the reverse step down exercise and progressing while working to improve form.

If the exercise is inappropriate to perform, first attempt the reverse step down exercise on a lower step but, if still inappropriate, then hold off on the lunge progression and work on half-kneeling balance if pain free.

How to progress or make harder: Raise the step height and/or add weight.

Half-Kneeling Balance

How to perform: Balance in a half kneeling position. Squeeze the glut and engage the core to open the hip and align the back hip and knee.

Additional information: In a proper half-kneeling stance, the front and back legs are in line, the knees are bent at 90 degrees, and the back hip is fully extended and aligned with the knee.

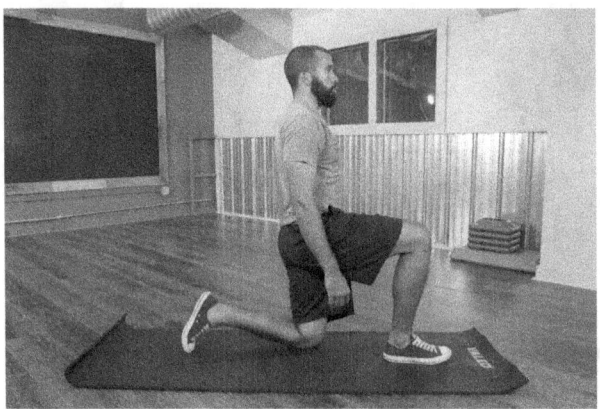

Both knees bent at 90 degrees, front and back feet in a straight line;
upright trunk;
back hip and knee aligned.

Ideal ability: Able to hold the position and balance for 30 seconds with perfect form and minimal difficulty.

Perfect form includes: Able to show good balance and control with no trunk movement. Both legs are in a straight line. Both knees are bent to 90 degrees. The back hip and knee are in perfect alignment and the back hip is fully extended.

BODY WEIGHT SQUAT PROGRESSION

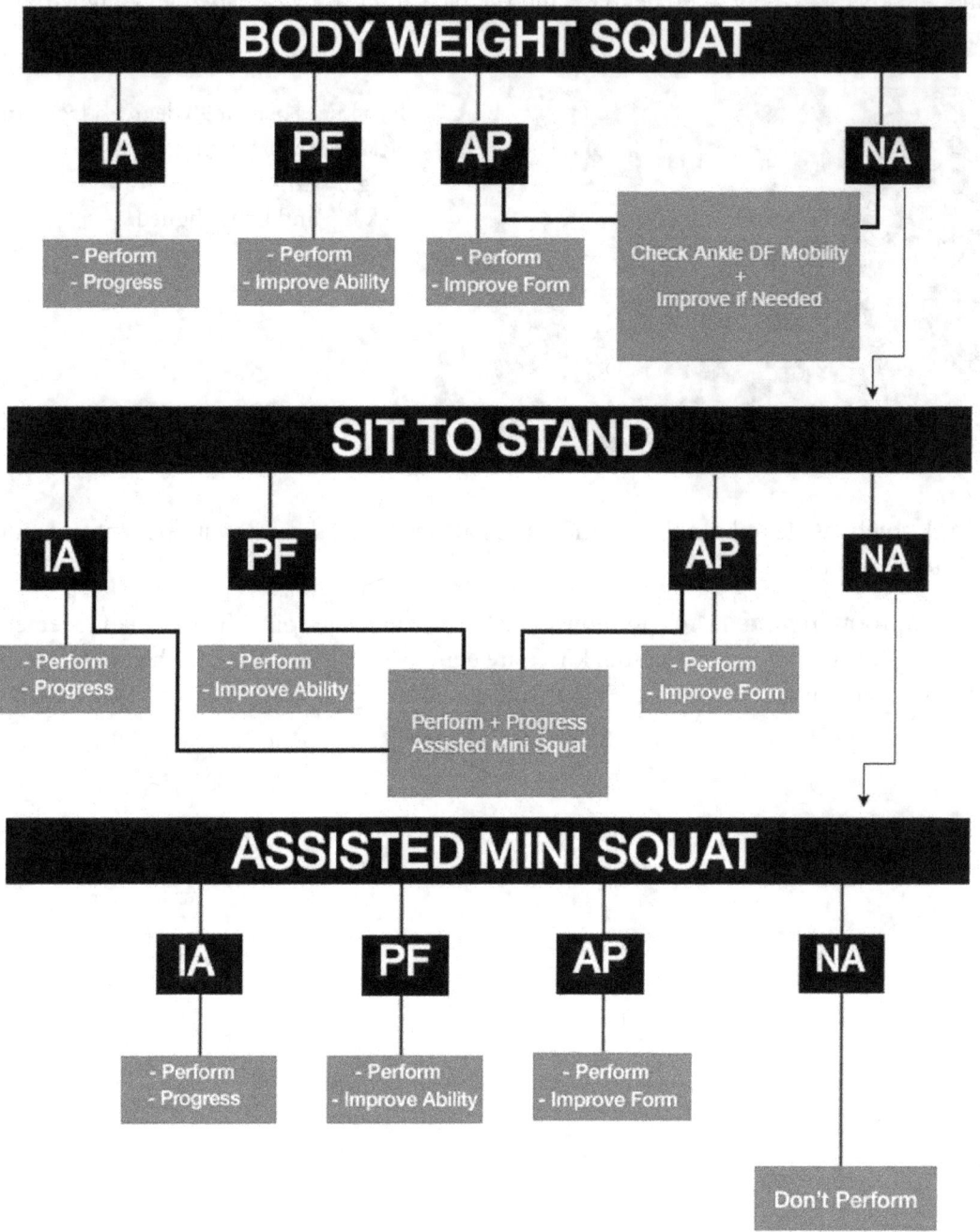

Body Weight Squat

How to perform: Stand with feet shoulder-width apart and toes facing forward. Sit the butt back and squat down with the hips slightly below horizontal. Stand back up, pushing the hips forward and squeezing the gluts at the top.

Additional information: Maintain an upright chest and neutral spine with the core engaged throughout. Push the knees outward slightly and don't allow the knees to go forward or collapse inward.

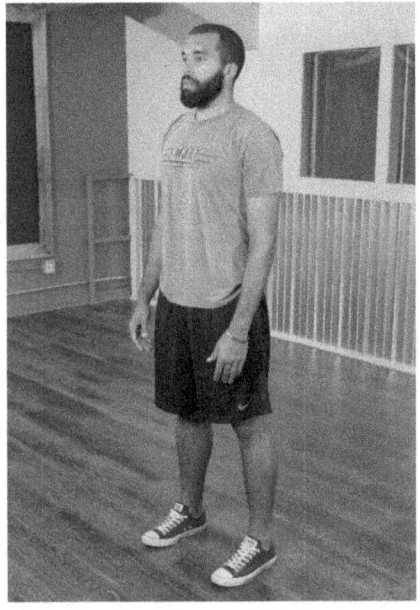 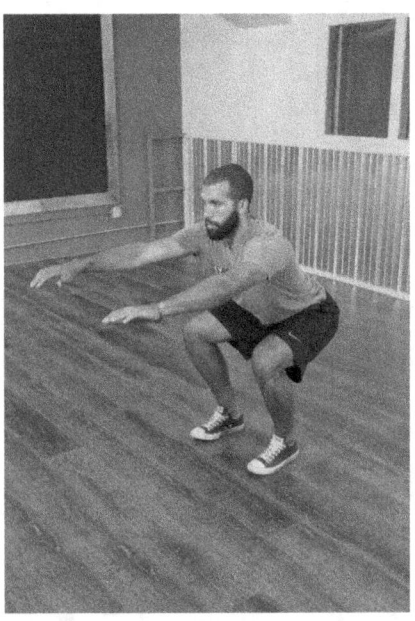

(a) Stand with feet shoulder width apart, toes facing forward;

(b) Lower into a squat.

Ideal ability: Able to complete a set of 20 repetitions with perfect form and minimal difficulty.

Perfect form includes: Able to squat down with the hips below horizontal and stand back up. Able to maintain a neutral spine throughout. The knees do not collapse inward or go forward.

Inappropriate to perform if: Unable to maintain a neutral spine throughout. Unable to prevent the knees from collapsing in or going forward past the toes, or causes pain.

If the body weight squat exercise is appropriate to perform but form requires improvement, continue performing the body weight squat exercise while working to improve form. Check ankle dorsi flexion mobility and, if limited, work to improve it (see *Mobility and Stretching* section for how to assess and improve ankle dorsi flexion mobility).

If the body weight squat exercise is inappropriate to perform, assess if the sit-to-stand exercise is appropriate to perform (assess using any seat height). Check ankle dorsi flexion mobility and, if limited, work to improve it (see *Mobility and Stretching* section for how to assess and improve ankle dorsi flexion mobility).

How to progress or make harder: Add weight and/or perform any variation of a single leg squat.

Sit-to-Stand

How to perform: Sit at the edge of a chair or sturdy object with the feet shoulder-width apart and the tibia (lower leg) in a vertical position. Lean forward hinging at the hips and stand up, pushing the hips forward and squeezing the gluts at the top. Then sit back down, slow and controlled.

Additional information: Maintain an upright chest and neutral spine with the core engaged throughout. Push the knees outward slightly; don't allow the knees to go forward or collapse inward.

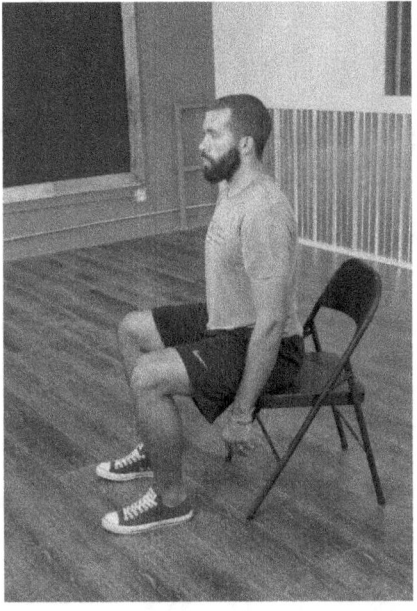 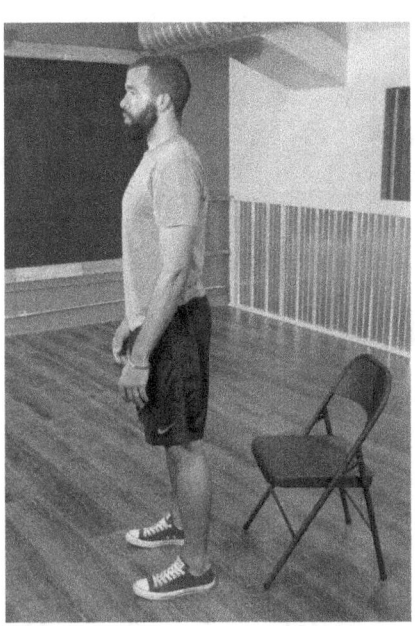

Sit with feet shoulder-width apart, toes facing forward, knees vertical;

(b) Stand up.

Ideal ability: Able to complete a set of 20 repetitions with perfect form and minimal difficulty (using a surface that places the hips at or below the knees in the seated position).

Perfect form includes: Able to show control while standing and sitting without plopping down. Able to maintain a neutral spine throughout. The knees do not collapse inward or go forward. The chest remains upright.

Inappropriate to perform if: Unable to maintain a neutral spine throughout. Unable to prevent the knees from collapsing in or going past the toes, or causes pain.

If the sit-to-stand exercise is appropriate to perform but form requires improvement, continue performing the sit-to-stand exercise while working to improve form. Slowly progress by lowering the seat height until the hips are below the knees in the seated position. Perform the assisted mini squat exercise and progress depth.

If the sit-to-stand exercise is inappropriate to perform, assess if the assisted mini squat exercise is appropriate to perform.

How to progress: Lower the seat height until thighs are below parallel. Tap the butt to the chair without sitting down completely. Add weight. Perform a single leg sit-to-stand.

Assisted Mini Squat

How to perform: Stand with feet shoulder-width apart and toes facing forward. Holding onto a sturdy object, sit the butt back and bend the knees slightly. Stand back up, pushing the hips forward and squeezing the gluts at the top.

Additional information: Maintain an upright chest and neutral spine with the core engaged throughout. Push the knees outward slightly and don't allow the knees to go forward or collapse inward.

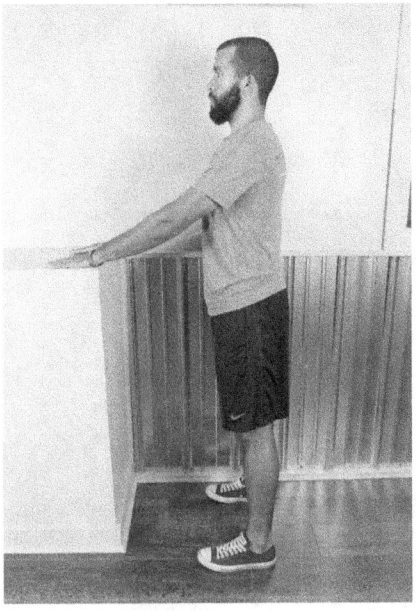

(a) Stand with feet shoulder-width apart, toes facing forward, holding a sturdy object;

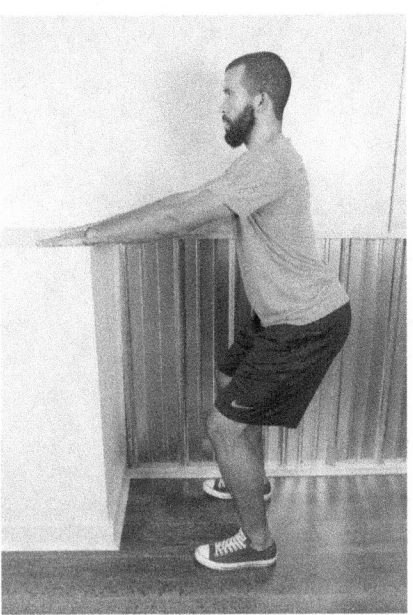

(b) Lower into a mini squat.

Ideal ability: Able to complete a set of 20 repetitions with perfect form and minimal difficulty.

Perfect form includes: Able to maintain a neutral spine throughout. The knees do not collapse inward or go forward. The chest remains upright.

Inappropriate to perform if: Unable to maintain a neutral spine throughout. Unable to prevent the knees from collapsing in or going past the toes, or causes pain.

If the assisted mini squat exercise is appropriate to perform but form requires improvement, continue performing the assisted mini squat exercise while progressing and working to improve form.

If the assisted mini squat exercise is inappropriate to perform, hold off on all squat activities.

How to progress: Lower the depth of the squat. Don't hold on (make sure form remains unchanged). Perform a single-leg assisted squat.

Postural and Upper Body Exercises

1. Band Row
2. Stability Ball I or Band Extension
3. Stability Ball T or
   Band Horizontal Abduction
4. Stability Ball Y
5. Side-Lying Shoulder External Rotation
   or Band Shoulder External Rotation
6. Band Shoulder Internal Rotation
7. Scaption Shoulder Raise
8. Overhead Press

Band Row

How to perform: Hold both ends of a band with the arms out straight and the palms facing each other. Squeeze the shoulder blades in and down and pull the arms straight back, bending the elbows and pause. Then, bring the arms back out with control.

Additional information: When pulling, bend the elbows to 90 degrees and keep the arms in close to the body. Avoid letting the shoulders shrug up.

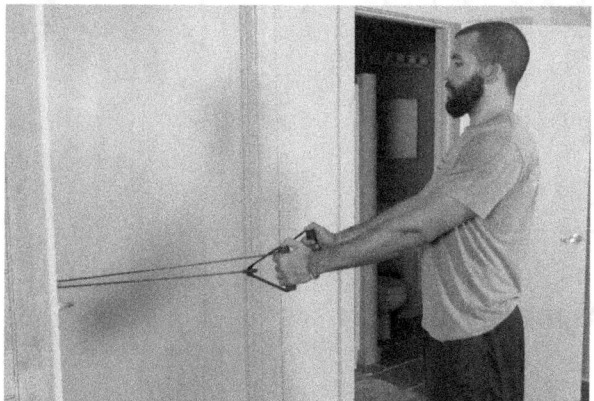

(a) Stand and hold both ends of a band with arms out in front;

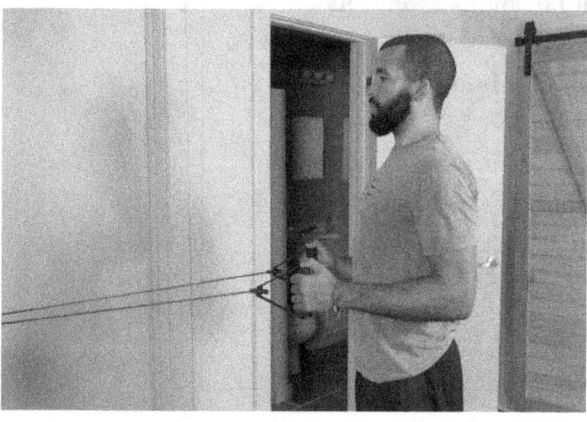

(b) Pull the arms straight back.

Ideal ability: Able to complete a set of 20 repetitions with perfect form and minimal difficulty using a medium tension band.

Perfect form includes: Arms are pulled straight back bringing the elbows slightly past the body and back out with control. The elbows stay close to the body and are bent to 90 degrees as the arms are pulled back. The shoulder blades are pulled in and down with no shoulder shrug.

How to progress: Use a heavier band or stand further away to create more resistance.

Stability Ball I

How to perform: Lie on your stomach on a stability ball with arms hanging straight down and the ball just below the rib cage. Squeeze the shoulder blades in and down and lift the arms straight back just above the height of the body. Pause at the top and lower back down with control.

Additional information: Maintain a neutral head position, and keep the elbows straight and palms facing down throughout.

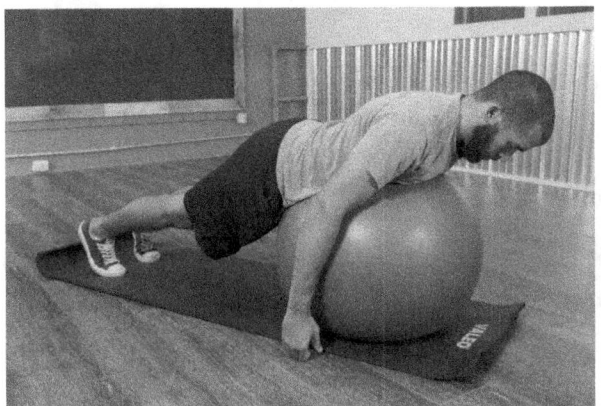

(a) Lie on your stomach on a stability ball with arms down;

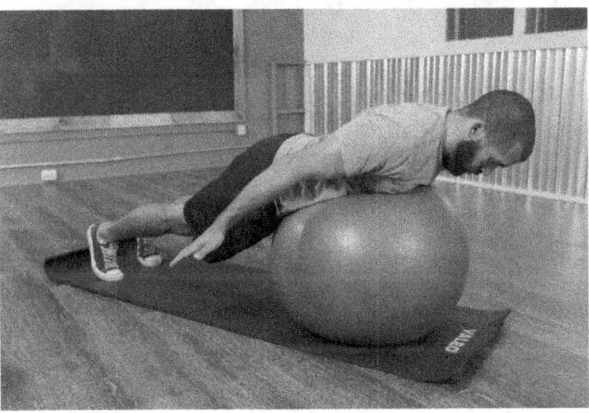

(b) Lift arms straight back and up.

Ideal ability: Able to complete a set of 20 repetitions with perfect form and minimal difficulty using a 5 lb. weight.

Perfect form includes: Arms are lifted just above the height of the body with the palms facing down and elbows straight. Shoulder blades are squeezed in and down during the movement and the shoulders don't shrug up.

How to progress: Add weight starting with 1 lb. and building up to 5 lbs.

If unable to perform with perfect form or the Stability Ball I exercise is uncomfortable, perform the band extension exercise.

Band Extension

How to perform: Hold both ends of a band with the arms out straight and the palms facing up. Squeeze the shoulder blades in and down and Pull the arms straight down to your side. Pause, then bring the arms back up with control.

Additional information: Keep the elbows straight and palms facing up throughout.

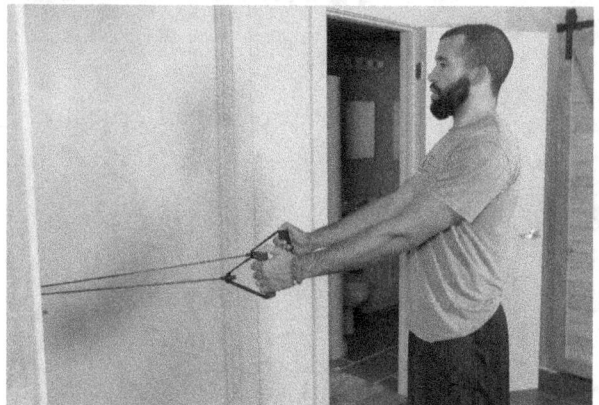

(a) Stand and hold both ends of a band with arms out in front;

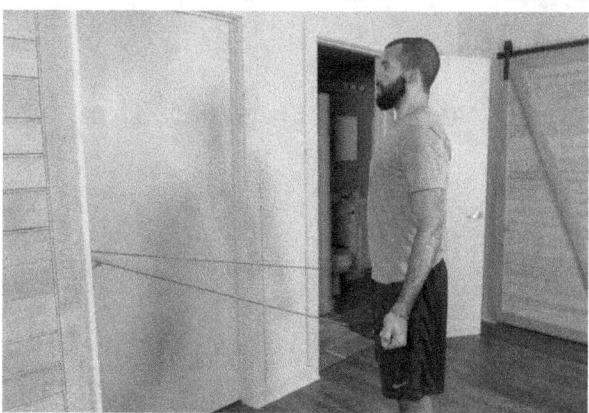

(b) Pull arms straight down and back.

Ideal ability: Able to complete a set of 20 repetitions with perfect form and minimal difficulty using a medium tension band.

Perfect form Includes: Arms are pulled straight back to the sides keeping the elbows straight and palms up. Shoulder blades are pulled in and down and shoulders don't shrug up.

How to progress: Use a heavier band or stand further back to create more resistance.

Stability Ball T

How to perform: Lie on your stomach on a stability ball with arms hanging straight down and the ball just below the rib cage. Squeeze the shoulder blades in and down and lift the arms straight out to the side to horizontal. Pause at the top and bring the arms back down with control.

Additional information: Maintain a neutral head position, and keep the elbows straight and thumbs facing up throughout.

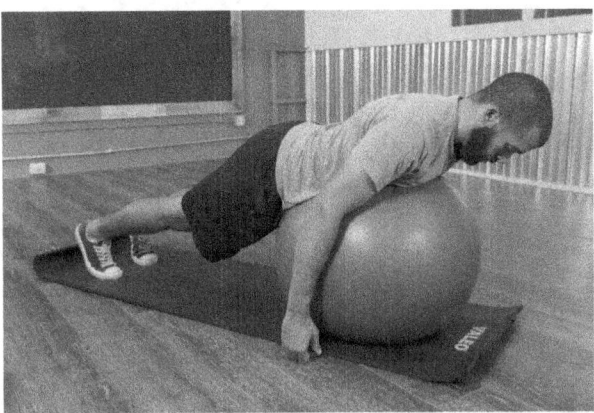

(a) Lie on your stomach on a stability ball with arms straight down;

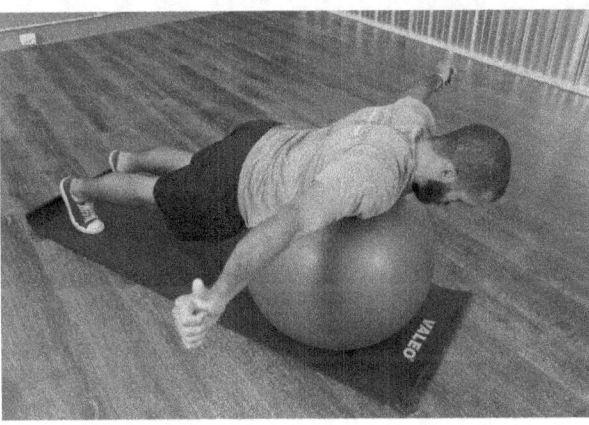

(b) Lift arms up straight out to the side.

Ideal ability: Able to complete a set of 20 repetitions with perfect form and minimal difficulty using a 5 lb. weight.

Perfect form includes: Arms are lifted directly out to the side with the elbows straight and thumbs facing up. Shoulder blades are squeezed in and down during the movement and the shoulders don't shrug up.

How to progress: Add weight starting with 1 lb. and building up to 5 lbs.

If unable to perform with perfect form or the stability ball T exercise is uncomfortable, perform the band horizontal abduction exercise.

Band Horizontal Abduction

How to perform: Hold both ends of a band with the arms out straight and the palms facing each other. Squeeze the shoulder blades in and down and pull the arms apart against the band. Pause at end range and bring the arms back together with control.

Additional information: Keep the elbows straight throughout.

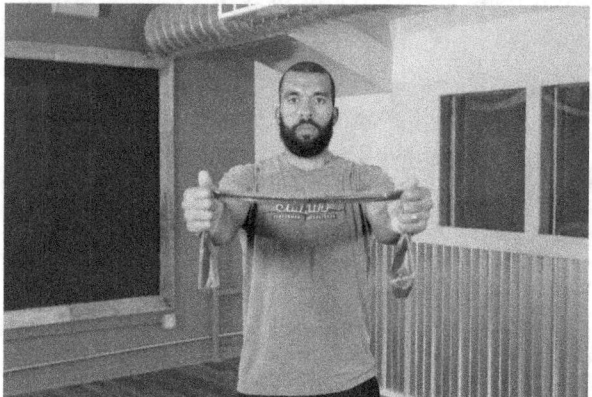

(a) Stand holding both ends of a band with arms straight out in front;

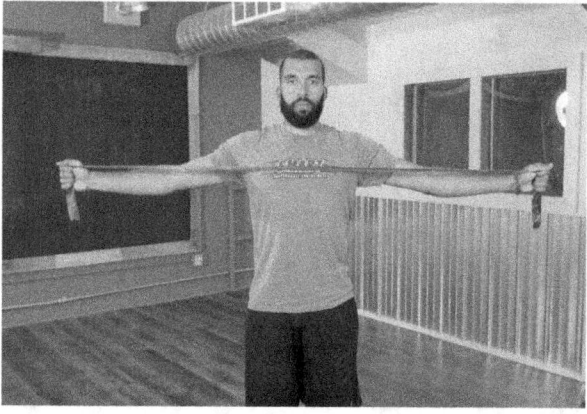

(b) Pull the arms apart.

Ideal ability: Able to complete a set of 20 repetitions with perfect form and minimal difficulty using a medium tension band.

Perfect form includes: Arms are pulled completely apart with the elbows straight and palms facing each other. Shoulder blades are squeezed in and down during the movement and the shoulders don't shrug up.

How to progress: Use a heavier band or start with the hands closer together on the band to create more resistance.

Stability Ball Y

How to perform: Lie on your stomach on a stability ball with arms hanging straight down and the ball just below the rib cage. Squeeze the shoulder blades in and down and lift the arms forward at a 45 degree angle to horizontal. Pause at the top and lower the arms back down with control.

Additional information: Maintain a neutral head position, and keep the elbows straight and thumbs facing up throughout.

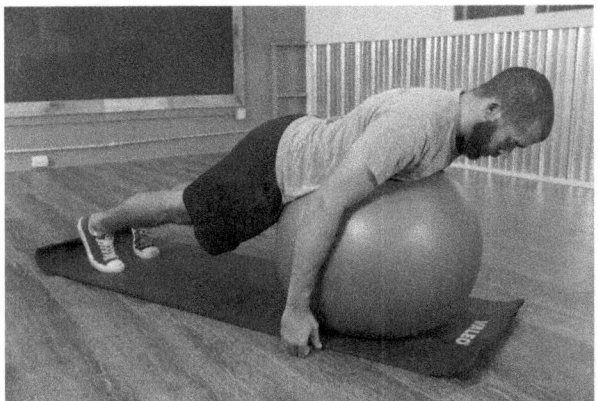

(a) Lie on your stomach on the stability ball with the arms straight down;

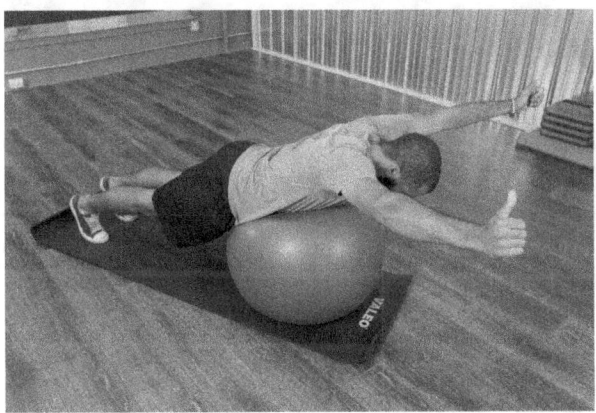

(b) Lift the arms up and out at a 45-degree angle.

Ideal ability: Able to complete a set of 20 repetitions with perfect form and minimal difficulty using 5 lb. weights.

Perfect form includes: Arms are lifted forward at a 45-degree angle to horizontal with the elbows straight and thumbs up.-Shoulder blades are squeezed in and down during the movement and the shoulders don't shrug up.

How to progress: Add weight starting with 1 lb. and building up to 5 lbs.

Side-Lying Shoulder External Rotation

How to perform: Grab a 1 to 5 lb. weight and lie on your side with the top arm flush to the body. Bend the elbow to 90 degrees and rest the hand on your belly. Squeeze the shoulder blade in and down and rotate the forearm slightly above horizontal. Pause at the top and lower the forearm back down with control.

Additional information: Keep the arm flush to the body and shoulder blade back and down throughout.

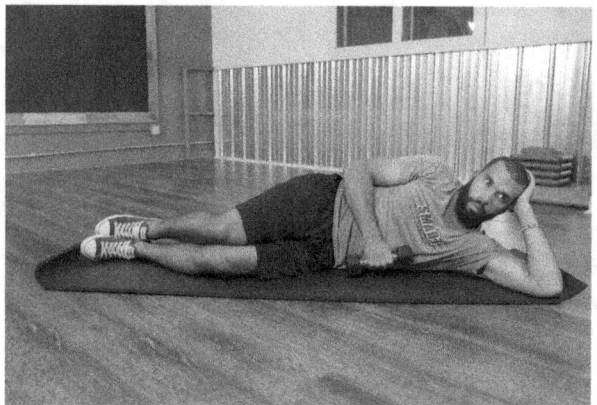

(a) Lie on your side with the arm flush to the body;

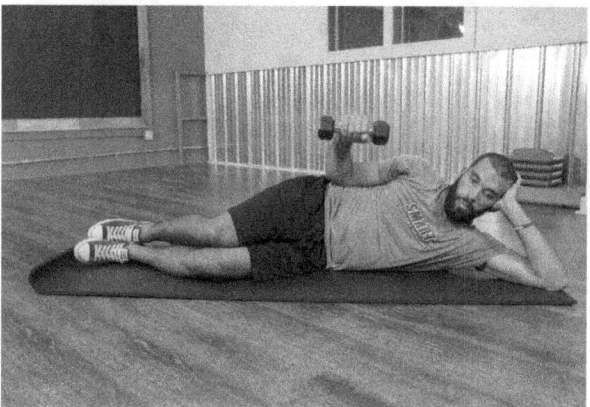

(b) Rotate the forearm upward.

Ideal ability: Able to complete a set of 20 repetitions on the right and left with perfect form and minimal difficulty using a 5 lb. weight.

Perfect form includes: The forearm rotates up just above horizontal and back down with control. Arm remains flush to the body with the elbow bent at 90 degrees. The shoulder stays back and down throughout and doesn't roll forward.

How to progress: Add weight, building up to 5 lbs.

Band Shoulder External Rotation

How to perform: Hold a band with the arm flush to the side, elbow bent to 90 degrees, and forearm resting on the belly. Squeeze the shoulder blade in and down and rotate the forearm out slightly past neutral. Pause at the end of the movement and bring the forearm back in with control.

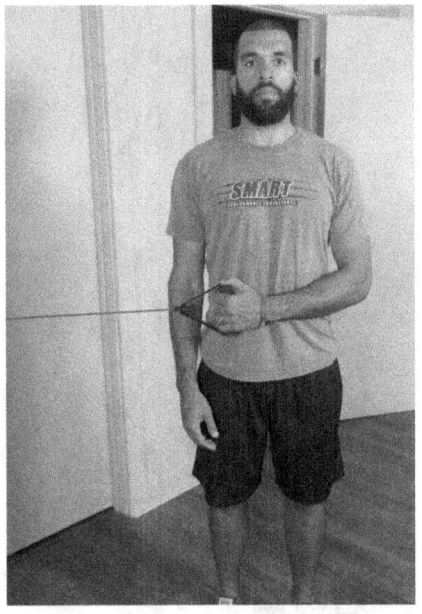 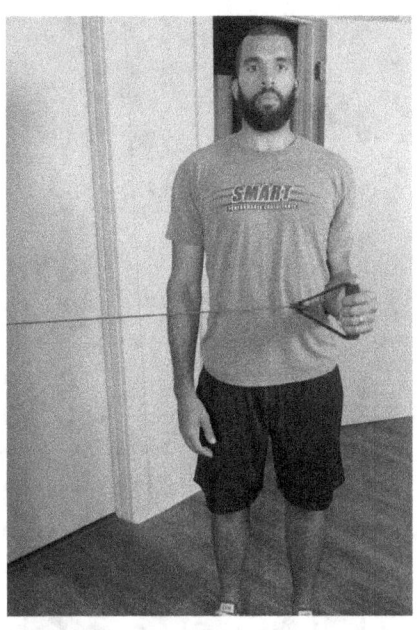

(a) Stand sideways holding a band with the arm flush to the body;

(b) Rotate the forearm out to the side.

Additional information: Keep the arm flush to the body and shoulder blade back and down throughout.

Ideal ability: Able to complete a set of 20 repetitions on the right and left with perfect form and minimal difficulty using a medium tension band.

Perfect form includes: The forearm rotates out just past neutral and back in with control. Arm remains flush to the body with the elbow bent at 90 degrees. The shoulder stays back and down throughout and doesn't roll forward.

How to progress: Use a tighter band or stand further away to create more resistance.

Band Shoulder Internal Rotation

How to perform: Hold a band with the arm flush to the side, elbow bent to 90 degrees and the forearm pointing out just past neutral. Squeeze the shoulder blade in and down and rotate the forearm in toward the belly; pause and bring the forearm back out.

Additional information: Keep the arm flush to the body and shoulder blade back and down throughout.

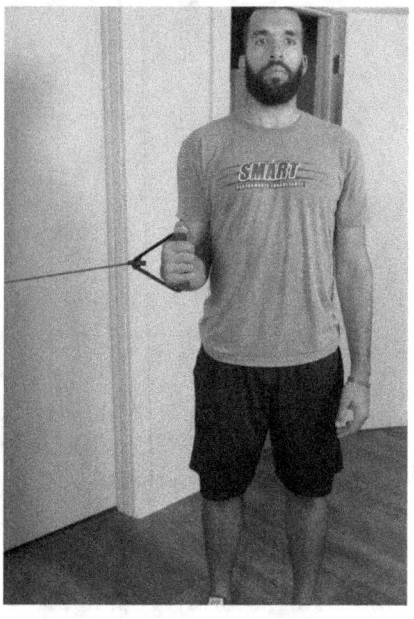

(a) Stand sideways holding a band with the arm flush to the body;

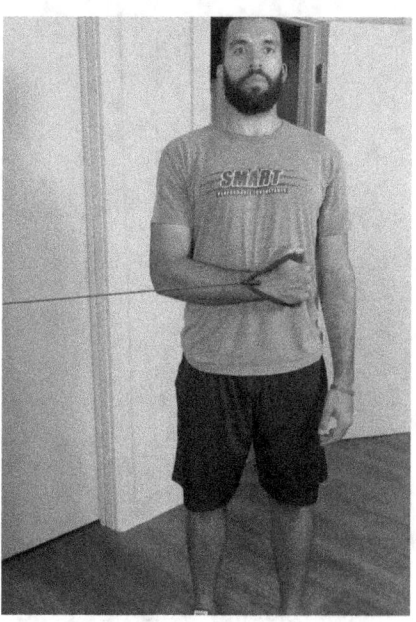

(b) Rotate the forearm in toward the stomach.

Ideal ability: Able to complete a set of 20 repetitions with perfect form and minimal difficulty using a medium tension band.

Perfect form includes: The forearm rotates in toward the belly and back out. Arm remains flush to the body with the elbow bent at 90 degrees. The shoulder stays back and down throughout and doesn't roll forward.

How to progress: Use a tighter band or stand further away to create more resistance.

Scaption Shoulder Raise

How to perform: Hold a 1 to 10 lb. weight in each hand and stand in a comfortable stance with the arms by the side. Lift the arms straight up at a 45-degree angle to shoulder height. Pause and lower the arms back down with control.

Additional information: Keep the elbows straight and avoid shrugging the shoulders.

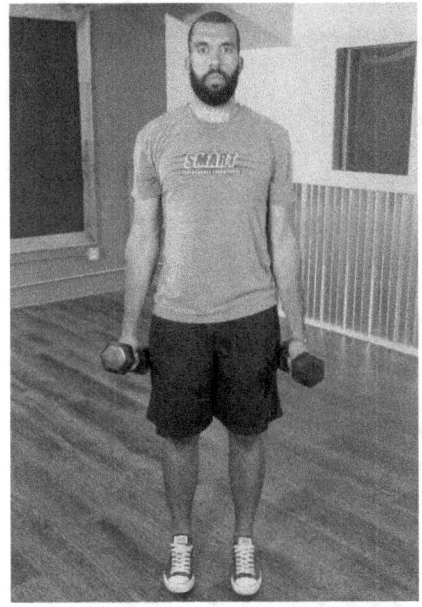

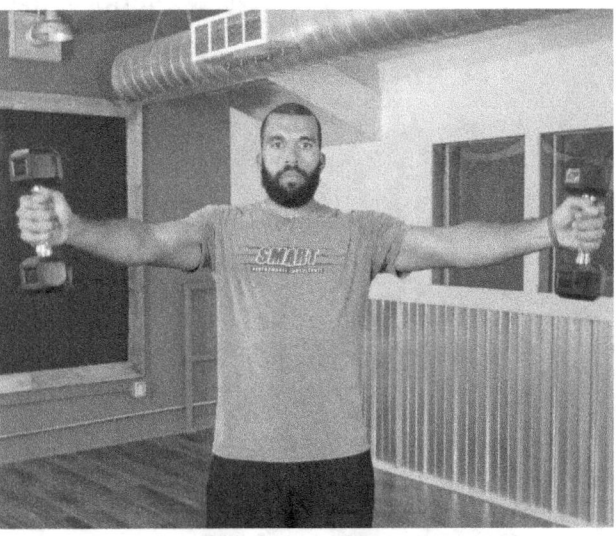

(b) Lift the arms up at a 45-degree angle.

(a) Hold weights with arms by your side;

Ideal ability: Able to complete a set of 20 repetitions with perfect form and minimal difficulty using a 10 lb. weight in each hand.

Perfect form includes: Arms are lifted up to shoulder height at a 45-degree angle with the elbows straight and thumbs up. The shoulders don't shrug up.

How to progress: Add weight, building up to 10 lbs.

Overhead Press

Criteria to be able to perform: Able to pass the wall shoulder flexion test. No shoulder pain with planks, side planks, push up, or any postural or upper body exercise.

How to perform the wall shoulder flexion test: Stand against a wall with your back flush to the wall. Lift your arms straight up trying to touch your thumbs to the wall.

Wall shoulder Flexion Test

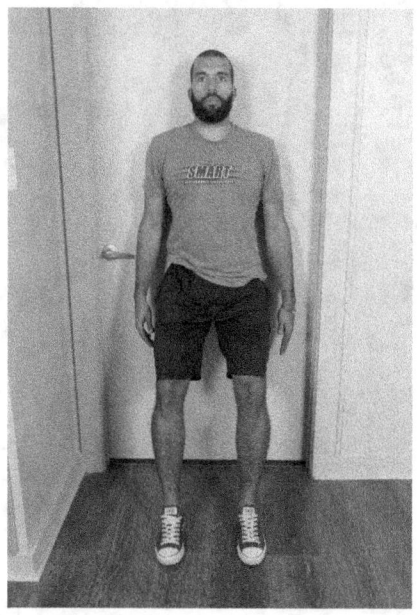 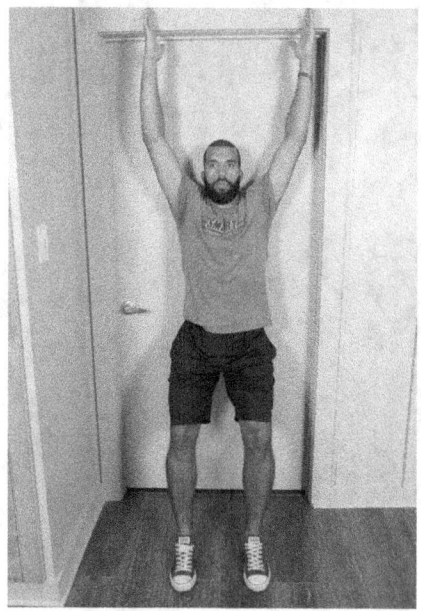

(a)Stand with the back flat against the wall and arms by your side;

(b) Lift the arms straight up to the wall.

Passing criteria: Able to touch the thumbs to the wall without the back losing contact with the wall or bending the elbows.

How to perform overhead press: Hold a 1 to 10 lb. weight in each hand and stand with feet shoulder-width apart; toes facing forward. Lift the hands to just above shoulder height with elbows bent and palms facing out. Push the arms straight up overhead; pause at the top and lower the arms back down with control.

Additional information: Avoid shrugging the shoulders or arching the back.

Overhead press

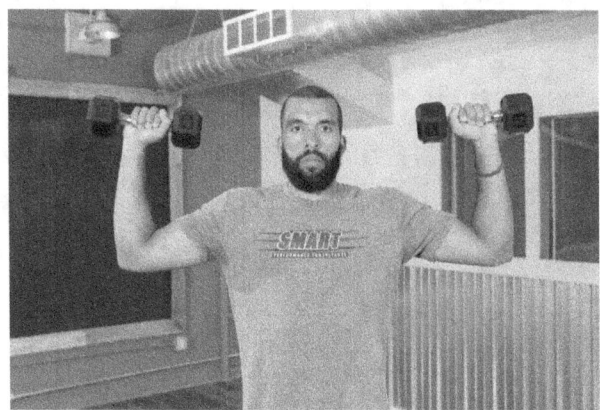

(a) Hands just above shoulder height;

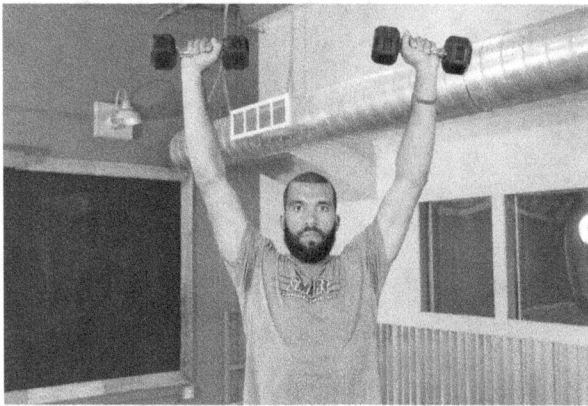

(b) Push the arms straight up.

Ideal ability: Able to complete a set of 20 repetitions with perfect form and minimal difficulty using 10 lb. weights.

Perfect form includes: Arms are fully extended over head with the elbows straight and the palms facing out; shoulders don't shrug up and the back doesn't arch.

How to progress: Add weight.

Mobility and Stretching

Stretching and mobility exercises help maintain and improve flexibility. They can also help normalize soft tissues and restore balance to muscles that have been overstressed with daily and recreational activities. For stretching to be effective, a person should fee a stretch in the muscle. The stretch should be light to medium intensity but should not be painful.

Soft tissue exercises such as foam rolling can be used in addition to stretching to improve and maintain mobility. For soft tissue exercises to be effective, a person should feel discomfort similar to when massaging a tight muscle. As the muscle loosens up, the amount of discomfort will decrease.

Additional information on stretching and mobility:

— Implement stretching and mobility exercises on a regular bases (minimum 2-3x a week) to improve and maintain good movement and physical health.
— Use stretching and mobility exercises to restore muscular balance and reduce post-exercise soreness following activity.
— Avoid prolonged static stretching prior to activity; instead use a dynamic warm up to increase blood flow and prepare the body for activity.
— If a muscle is knotted up, foam roll or massage the muscle first before stretching it.

Stretches, Foam Roll Exercises, and Mobility Tests

Stretches, mobility exercises, and mobility tests that assess and/or improve:

Ankle mobility:

→ Runners' stretch (straight and bent knee)
→ Ankle wall dorsi flexion mobility test
→ Foam roll calf

Hamstring mobility:

→ Wall hamstring stretch
→ Strap hamstring stretch
→ Foam roll hamstring

Hip flexor and quad mobility:

→ Prone quad stretch
→ Half-kneeling hip flexor stretch
→ Foam roll quad, hip flexor, and ITB

Glut mobility:

→ Standing pigeon stretch
→ Figure-4 glut stretch
→ Foam roll glut

Groin/adductor mobility:

→ Straddle stretch

Low back extension mobility:

→ Prone press up:

Low back flexion mobility:

→ Prayer stretch
→ Seated chair flexion stretch
→ Double knees-to-chest stretch
→ Single knee-to-chest stretch

Shoulder flexion mobility:

→ Stick shoulder flexion stretch
→ Wall shoulder flexion stretch

Shoulder internal rotation mobility:

→ Sleeper shoulder internal rotation stretch
→ Strap functional shoulder internal rotation

Anterior chest mobility:

→ Corner or doorway pec stretch
→ Foam roll pec stretch

Thoracic spine mobility:

→ Thoracic spine foam roll extension
→ Thoracic spine foam roll extension with arms overhead
→ Thoracic spine foam roll extension with weight and arms overhead
→ Foam roll thoracic spine

Runners' Stretch

How to perform (with straight knee): Stand with feet together, toes facing forward, with the hands resting on a wall or sturdy object. Step back with the foot you are stretching. Bend the front knee and lean into the stretch and hold.

How to perform (with bent knee): Same set up as with straight knee but instead of keeping the back knee straight, bend the back knee. Pause 3 to 5 seconds and straighten the knee out.

Additional information: Keep the back foot straight and the heel flat on the floor.

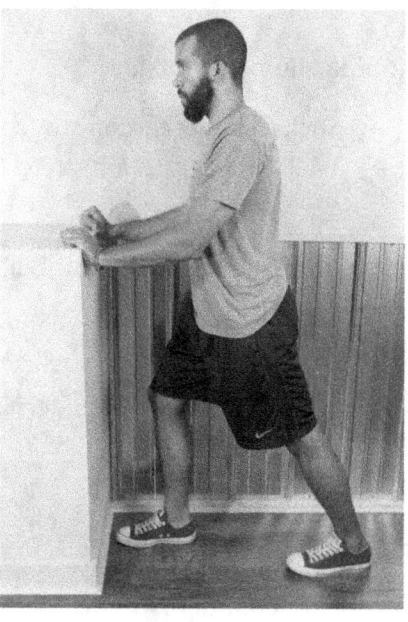
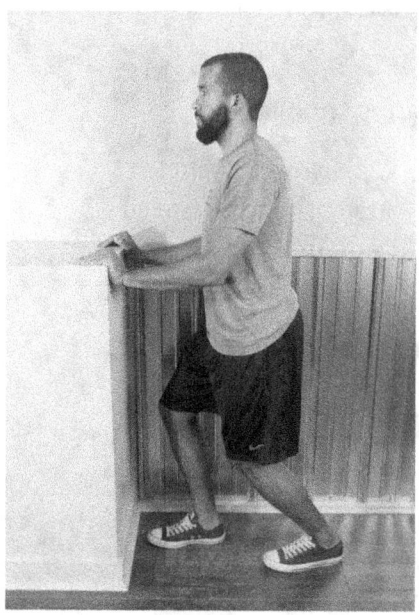

(a) Back knee straight.   (b) Back knee bent.

Ankle Wall Dorsi Flexion Mobility Test

How to perform: Stand with feet together, toes facing forward, with the hands resting on a wall. Place the foot you are assessing one fist length way from the wall. Bend the front knee and try to touch the knee to the wall while keeping the heel on the floor.

Additional information: Keep the foot you are assessing straight.

Ideal mobility: Able to touch the knee to the wall, keeping the heel flat on the floor, with the foot one fist length away from the wall.

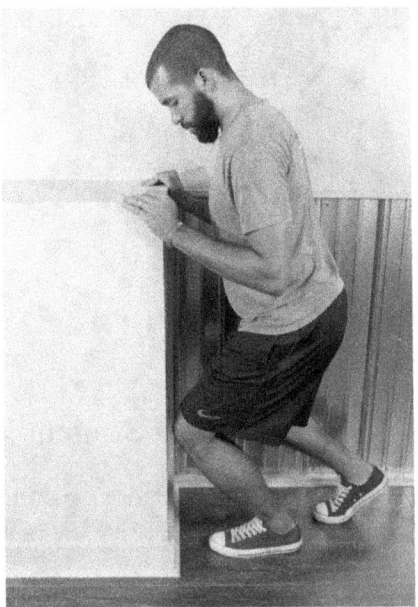

Knee touching wall.

Foam Roll Calf

How to perform: Place a foam roll under the ankle and cross the other foot over. Use the upper body to roll back and forth over the foam roll trying to hit all parts of the calf muscle. The calf runs from the ankle to the knee.

Additional information: Search for tight areas by rotating the leg right and left. If you find a tight area stay in that spot until it loosens up.

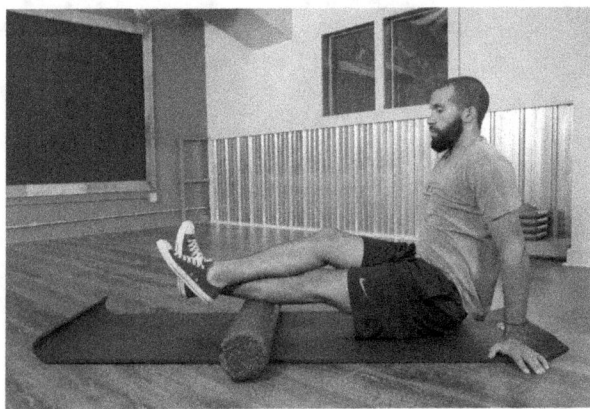

Roll back and forth over the calf and lower leg.

Wall Hamstring Stretch

How to perform: Lie on your back and prop one foot up on the wall with the other flat on the floor. Scoot forward towards the wall as far as you can, keeping both knees straight and hold.

Additional information: Keep both knees straight and don't allow the bottom foot to turn out.

Ideal mobility: Able to scoot forward so the leg is flush to the wall and the foot is pointing straight up while keeping both knees straight.

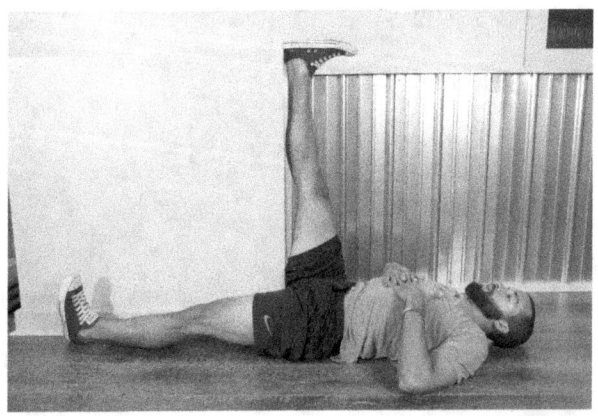

Leg flush to the wall, foot pointing straight up.

Strap Hamstring Stretch

How to perform: Loop a strap around one foot and lie on your back. Slowly lift the leg pulling with the strap as far as you can while keeping both knees straight and hold.

Additional information: Keep both legs straight and don't allow the bottom foot to turn out.

Ideal mobility: Able to lift the leg to 90 degrees, pointing the foot straight up while keeping both knees straight.

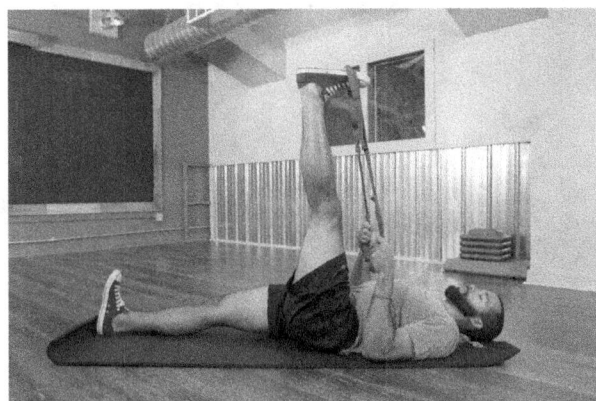

Lift leg to 90 degrees.

Foam Roll Hamstring

How to perform: Place a foam roll under the thigh and cross the other foot over. Use the upper body and roll back and forth over the foam roll trying to hit the hamstring muscle. The hamstring runs from the knee to the butt.

Additional information: Search for tight areas by rotating the leg right and left. If you find a tight area stay in that spot until it loosens up.

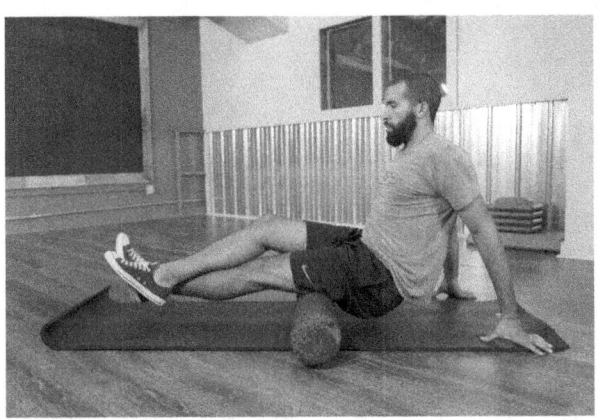

Roll back and forth over the hamstring.

Prone Quad Stretch

How to perform: Lie on your stomach with your feet together and legs straight. Bend one knee and grab your foot, trying to touch the heel to the butt.

Additional information: Keep both hips flat on the floor and you do not rotate to one side. If you're unable to grab the foot, use a strap to pull.

Ideal mobility: Able to touch the heel to the butt keeping both hips flat on the floor.

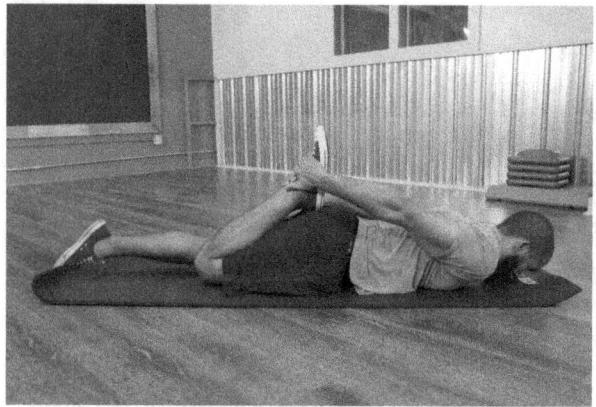

(a) Pull the heel to butt.

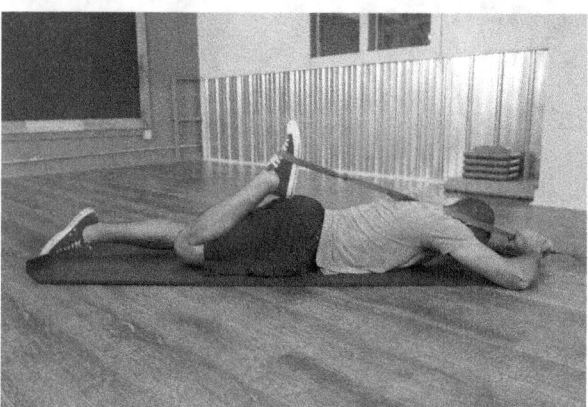

(b) Pull the heel to butt, using a strap.

Half-Kneeling Hip Flexor Stretch

How to perform: Get into a half-kneeling position with both knees bent at 90 degrees. Squeeze the back glut, tilt the pelvis underneath, and push the back hip forward and hold.

Additional information: Maintain an upright trunk and neutral low back position. Keep the front knee vertical and don't allow it to go forward past the toes.

Ideal mobility: Able to achieve full hip extension with an upright trunk and neutral spine.

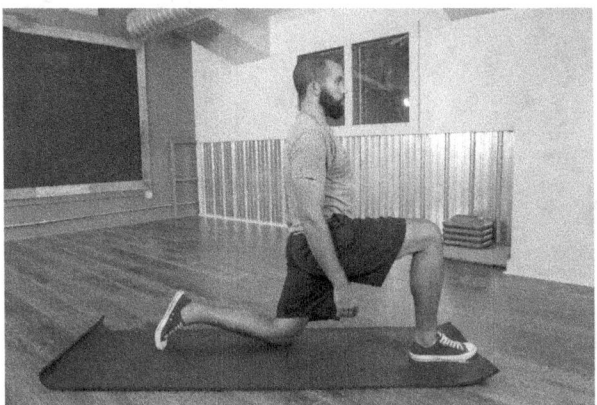

Squeeze the glut, tuck the pelvis underneath, and push the back hip forward.

Foam Roll Quad and Hip Flexor

How to perform: Lie on your stomach and place the foam roll under the hip and thigh. Use the upper body and other leg to roll back and forth over the foam roll, trying to hit the hip flexor and quad muscles. The hip flexor and quad runs from the knee to the hip.

Additional information: Search for tight areas by rotating the leg right and left. If you find a tight area, stay in that spot until it loosens up.

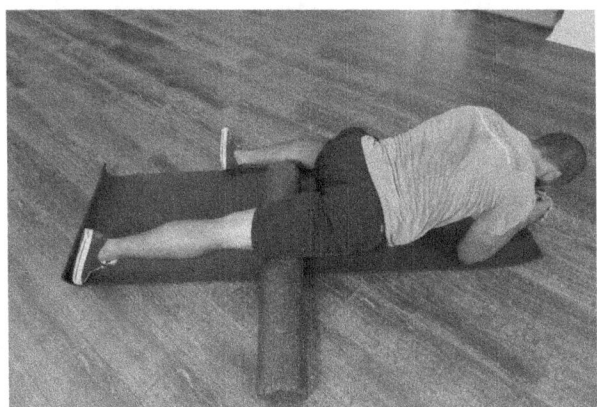

Roll back and forth over the quad and hip flexor.

Foam Roll ITB

How to perform: Lie on your side and place the foam roll under the down thigh and cross the other leg over placing the foot on the ground. Use the upper body and leg to roll back and forth over the foam roll trying to hit the ITB. The ITB runs from the hip to the knee.

Additional information: Search for tight areas by rotating the leg right and left. If you find a tight area stay in that spot until it loosens up.

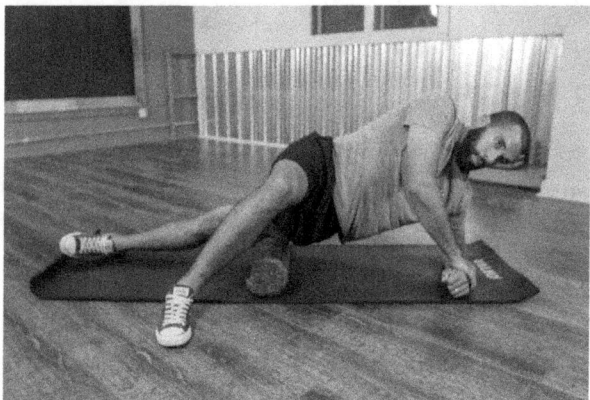

Roll back and forth over the IT band.

Standing Pigeon Stretch

How to perform: Stand in front of a flat surface about thigh high. Place one leg up on the surface with the knee bent and the thigh pointing straight ahead perpendicular to the body. Try to push the knee flush to the surface and hinge forward at the hips trying to rest the ribcage on the thigh and hold.

Additional information: Maintain a neutral spine position throughout.

Ideal mobility: Able to rest the ribcage on the thigh with the knee flush to the table.

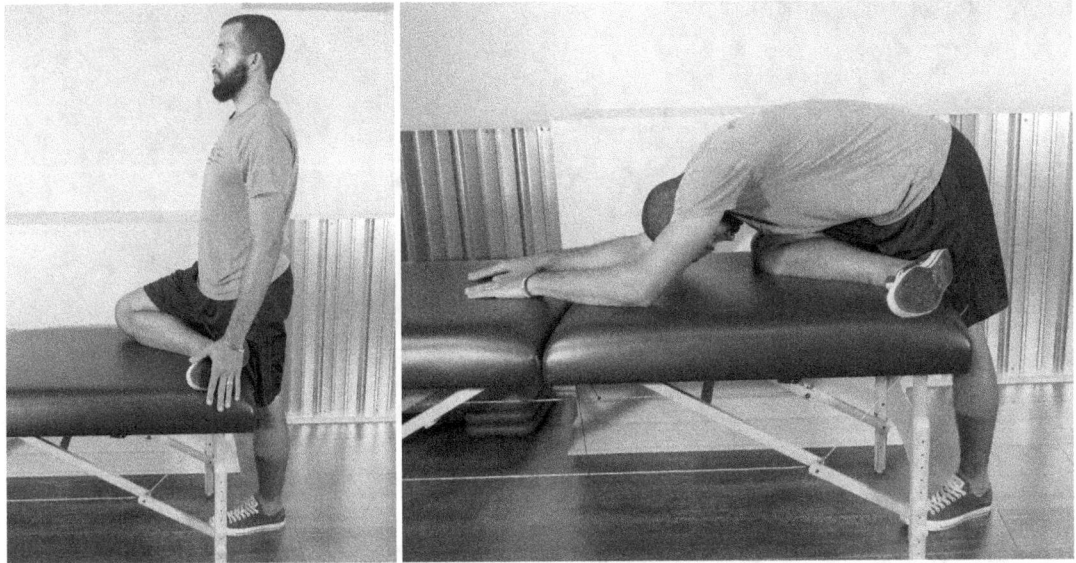

Push knee flush to the surface; rest the ribcage on the thigh.

Figure-4 Glut Stretch

How to perform: Lie on your back with the knees bent up. Cross the foot you're stretching over the other knee and slowly flex the knee up, pulling with the hands until you feel a stretch and hold.

Additional information: If you can't reach the thigh to pull, you can use a strap.

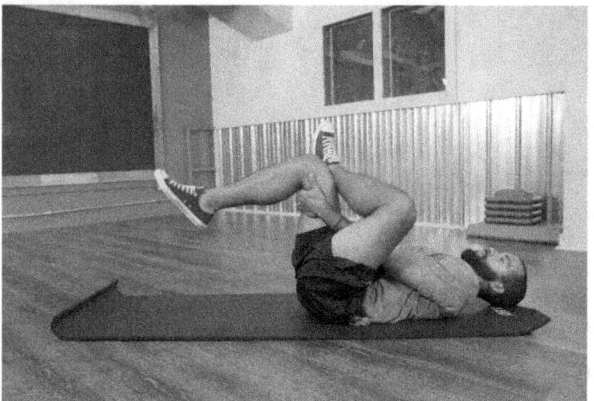

(a) Pull thigh up with foot crossed.

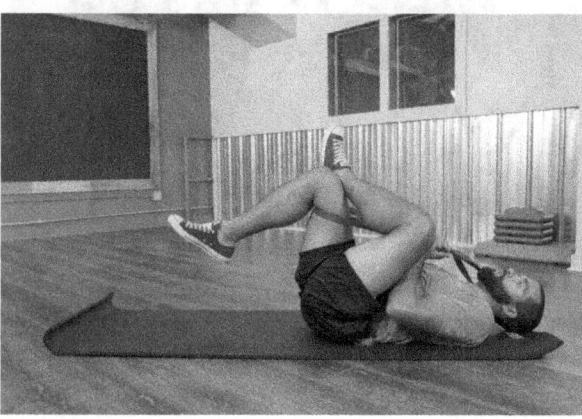

(b) Pull thigh up with foot crossed using a strap.

Foam Roll Glut

How to perform: Sit on the foam roll and cross the leg your stretching over the knee. Lean slightly to the side you are stretching and use the upper body and other leg to roll back and forth over the foam roll trying the hit the glut muscle.

Additional information: Search for tight areas by leaning to the right and the left. If you find a tight area stay in that spot until it loosens up.

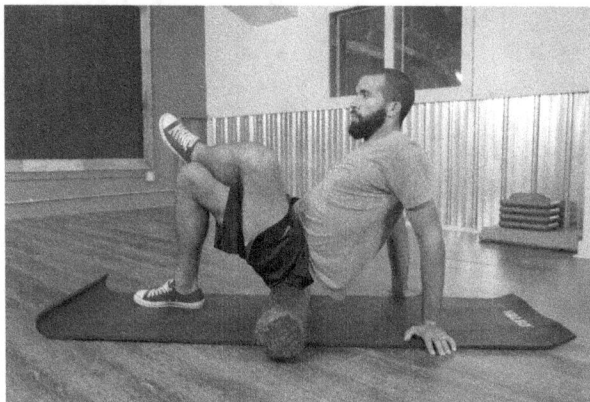

Roll back and forth over the glut.

Straddle Stretch

How to perform: Sit in a straddle position with the knees straight and reach the hands forward, hinging at the hips and hold.

Additional information: Maintain a neutral spine.

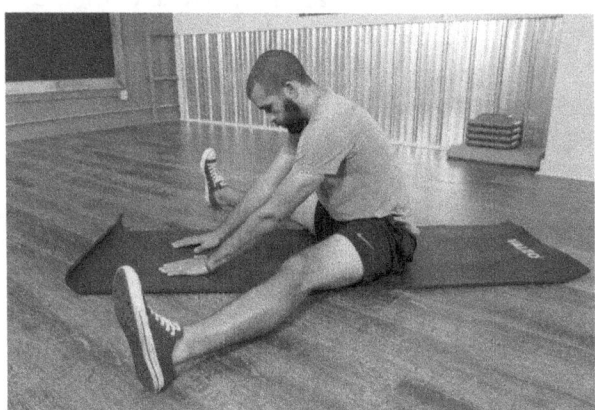

Reach the arms forward hinging at the hips.

Prone Press Up

How to perform: Lie on your stomach with your hands just above your shoulders. Push the arms as straight as you can while keeping the hips on the floor. Pause at the top and come back down.

Ideal mobility: Able to push arms straight with hips on the floor.

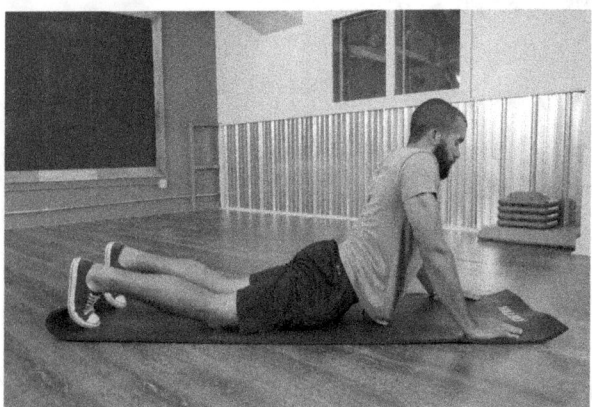

Push arms straight with hips on the floor.

Prayer Stretch

How to perform: Get on all fours, then sit back on the heels and reach the hands forward, trying to rest the ribcage on the thighs and hold.

Ideal mobility: Able to rest the rib cage on the thigh.

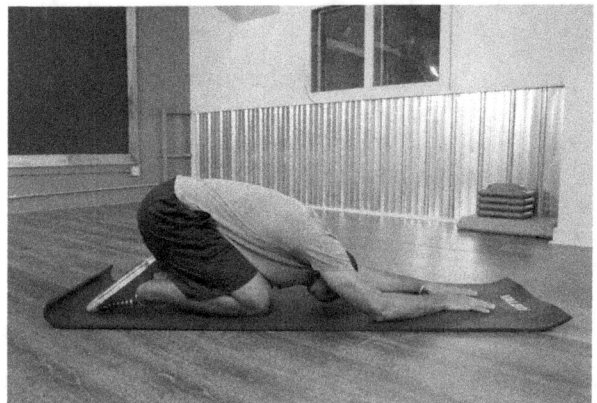

Reach the hands forward and rest the ribcage on thighs.

Seated Chair Flexion Stretch

How to perform: Sit at the edge of a chair with your knees and feet wider than shoulder width. Bend forward, reaching your hands to the ground. Pause 3 to 5 seconds and come back up.

Additional information: Relax at the bottom of the stretch and don't force more motion than what is comfortable.

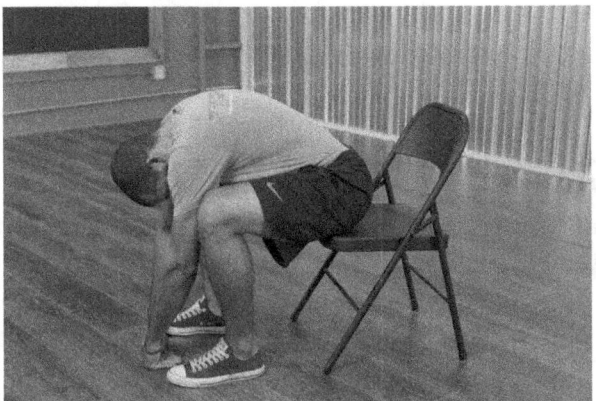

Bend forward, reaching hands to the floor.

Double Knees-To-Chest Stretch

How to perform: Lie on your back with the knees bent up. Lift your knees up and pull them to the chest as far as you can. Pause 3 to 5 seconds and lower the legs back down.

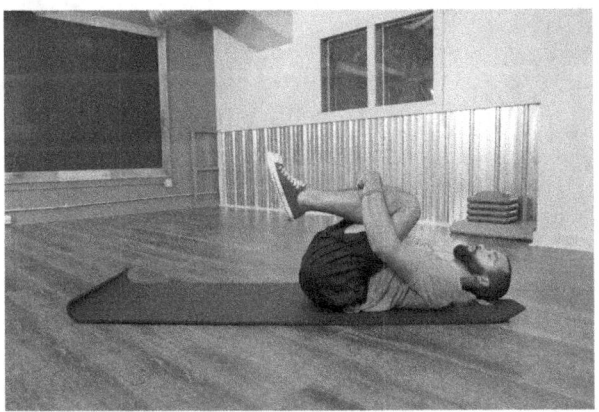

Pull knees to chest.

Single Knee-To-Chest Stretch

How to perform: Lie on your back with one leg bent up and the other straight. Lift the bent knee up and pull it to the chest. Pause 3 to 5 seconds and lower the leg back down.

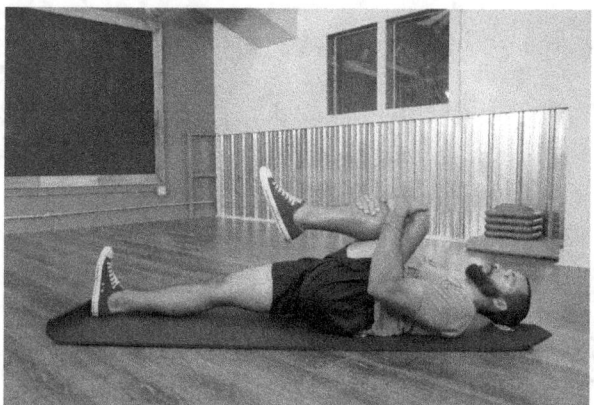

Pull the knee to chest.

Stick Shoulder Flexion Stretch

How to perform: Lie on your back. Hold a stick with the hands shoulder-width apart and lift the arms overhead, keeping the elbows straight and hold.

Additional information: Keep the lower back flat to the floor.

Ideal mobility: Able to touch the backs of the hands to the floor with hands shoulder-width apart and lower back flat to the floor.

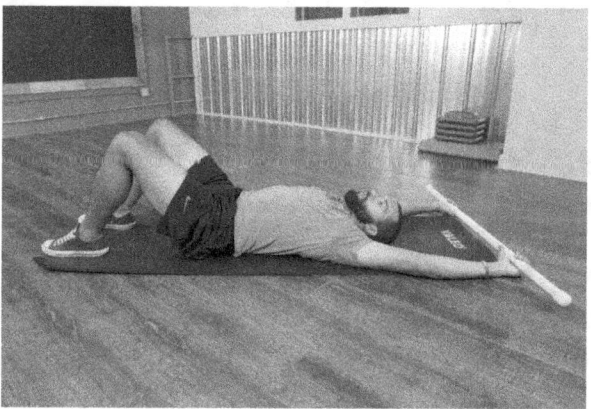

Hands shoulder-width apart, lift arms overhead touching the floor.

Wall Shoulder Flexion Stretch

How to perform: Stand in a doorway and reach one arm straight up, resting it on the wall. Step forward with the same leg and lean into the stretch, trying to push the armpit forward and hold.

Additional information: Keep the arm straight and maintain a neutral low back position.

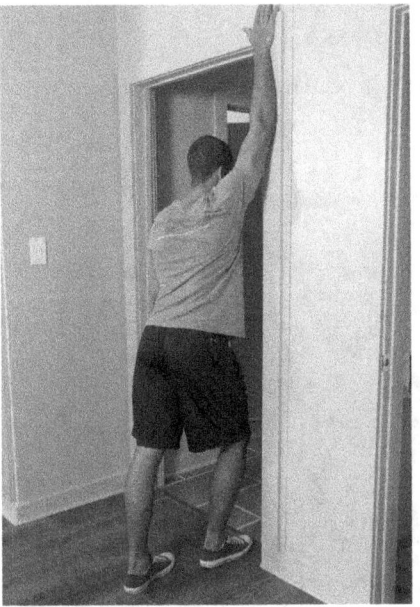

Reach arm up on wall and push armpit forward.

Sleeper Shoulder Internal Rotation Stretch

How to perform: Lie on your side with the bottom arm perpendicular to the body and the elbow bent to 90 degrees. Roll backward slightly so the shoulder blade is flush to the floor. Use the other hand to rotate the forearm down trying to touch the palm to the floor and hold.

Additional information: Keep the shoulder blade in contact with the floor and avoid letting the shoulder roll forward.

Ideal mobility: Able to rotate forearm so the hand is approximately a fist length from the floor keeping the shoulder blade flush to the floor.

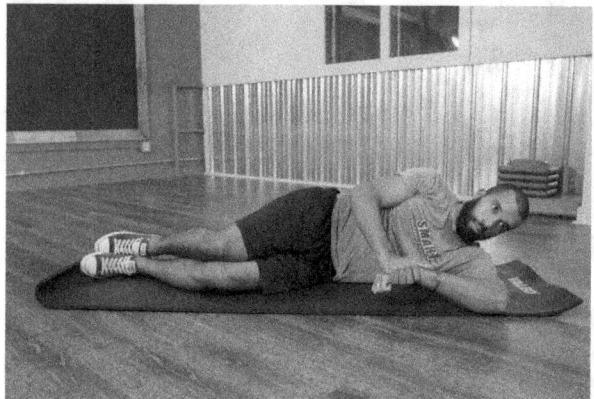

Rotate forearm down toward the ground.

Strap Functional Shoulder Internal Rotation Stretch

How to perform: Reach and pull the one hand up the back using a strap. Pause 3 to 5 seconds and let the hand come back down.

Additional information: Maintain an upright posture and avoid letting the shoulder roll forward.

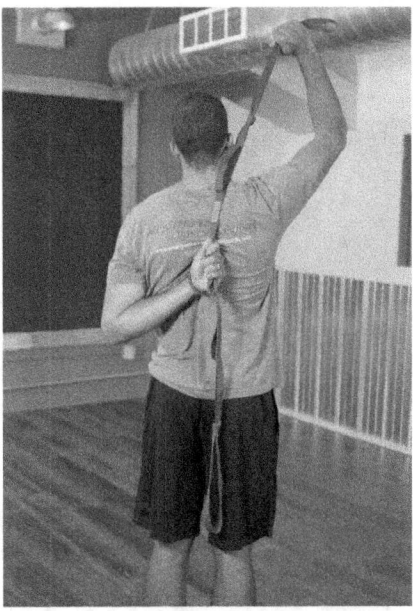

Reach and pull the hand up the back using the strap.

Ideal mobility: Able to touch the opposite shoulder blade without rolling the shoulder forward and maintaining an upright posture.

Corner or Doorway Pec Stretch

How to perform: Stand in front of a corner or doorway. Place both arms up on the wall just below shoulder height with the elbows bent at a 90-degree angle and the forearms flush against the wall. Step forward with either foot and bend the front knee to lean into the stretch and hold.

Additional information: Relax the arms and control the stretch with the front leg.

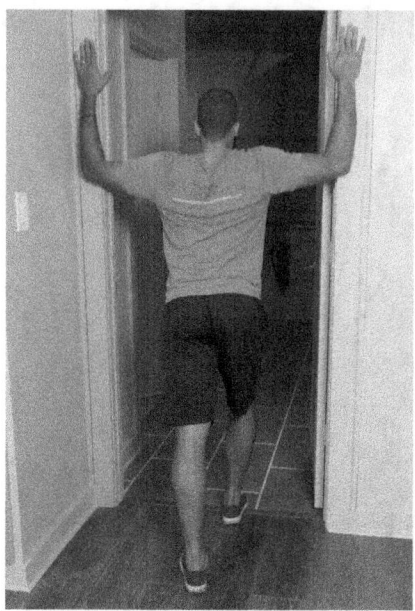

Place arms on the wall and lean forward, pushing the chest forward.

Foam Roll Pec Stretch

How to perform: Lie on your back with the foam roll resting between the shoulder blades and arms out to the side.

Additional information: Keep the palms facing up.

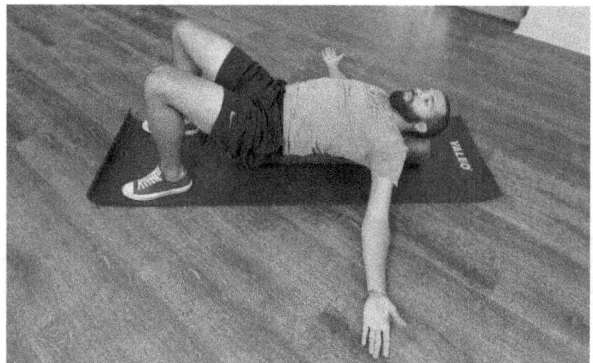

Lie over the foam roll with the arms out to the side.

Thoracic Spine Foam Roll Extension

How to perform: Lie on your back over a foam roll with the roll just below the shoulder blades. Cross the hands behind the head and extend over the foam roll. Pause 3 to 5 seconds and come back up.

Additional information: The foam roll can be positioned higher or lower in the thoracic spine depending on where tightness is felt.

To progress: Perform the stretch with arms overhead.

For an even greater stretch: Lift the hips up and reach the arms overhead grabbing a weight, then drop the hips extending the upper back over the foam roll. Pause 3 to 5 seconds and lift the hips back up.

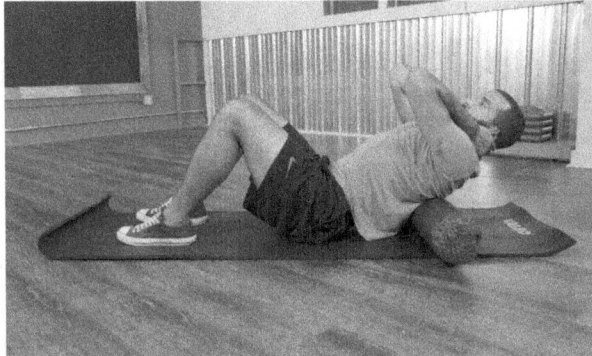

T spine foam roll extension
(a) Extend over the foam roll;

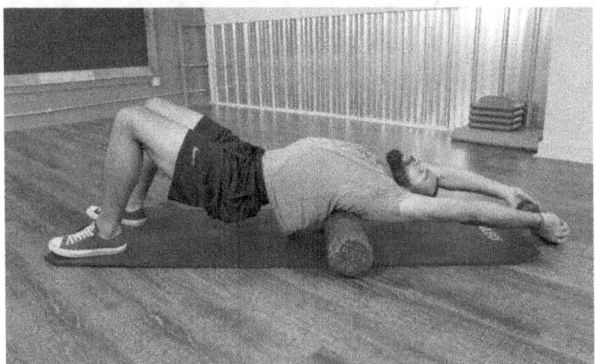

T spine foam roll extension with arms overhead
(b) Reach arms over head and extend over the foam roll;

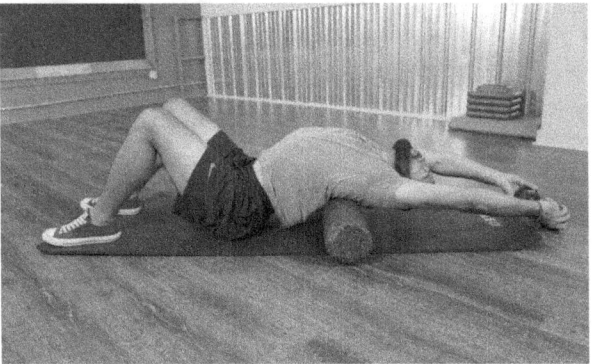

T spine foam roll extension with weight and arms overhead
(c) Reach arms over head, grabbing a weight and lift hips up; then drop the hips, extending over the foam roll.

Foam Roll Thoracic Spine

How to perform: Lie on your back over a foam roll with the foam roll resting just below the shoulder blades. Cross the hands behind the head and roll back and forth over the foam roll trying to hit the area of the thoracic spine. The thoracic spine runs from the bottom of the neck to just below the shoulder blades.

Additional information: Search for tight areas by rotating the trunk slightly to the left and the right. If you find a tight area, stay in that spot until it loosens up.

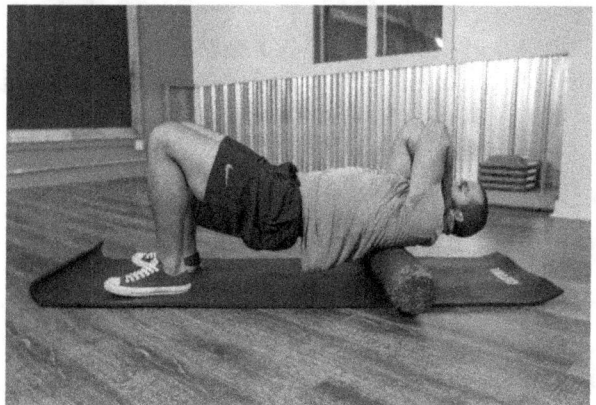

Roll back and forth over the thoracic spine.

Running and Jumping

The ability to run and jump is foundational to human movement and is required for many recreational activities. Jogging, jump rope, and other exercises involving jumping are also great ways to maintain and improve cardiovascular health. However, before engaging in activities that involve running and jumping, a person should have the basic skills to perform the activities safely.

Criteria for Running and Jumping

1. Able to perform 10 single leg heel raises on the right and left.
2. Able to perform 20 double leg jumps on the balls of the feet without the heels touching.
3. Able to perform 20 steps jogging in place on the balls of the feet without the heels touching.
4. Able to perform 5 mini squat jumps showing proper jumping and landing mechanics.
5. Able to perform 20 heel taps off a 6-inch step on the right and left.
6. No pain with above criteria.
7. No pain with any foundational movement or exercise.

Single Leg Heel Raises

How to perform: Stand on one leg and push up onto the ball of the foot lifting the heel and foot off the ground; then slowly lower back down

Additional information: You can hold onto a sturdy object or wall for balance

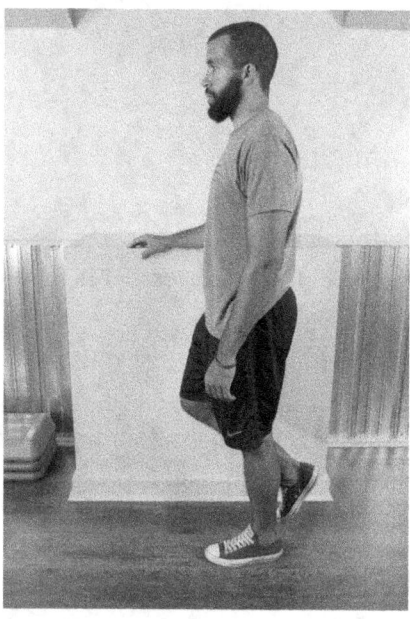

(a) Stand on one leg;

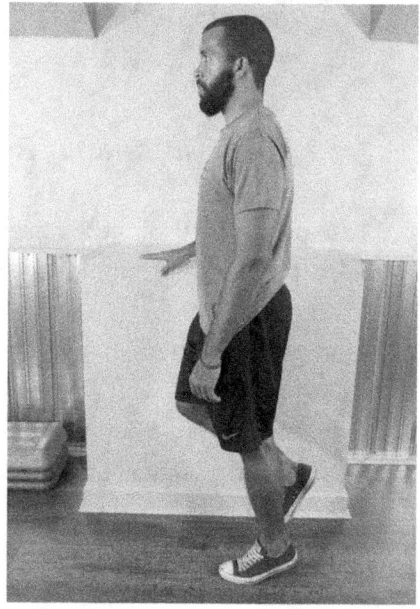

(b) Push up on the ball of the foot, lifting the heel off the ground.

Double Leg Jumping on the Balls of the Feet

How to perform: Stand with feet close together and jump up and down on the balls of your feet without letting the heels touch the ground.

Additional information: Maintain a soft landing and do not lock out the knees.

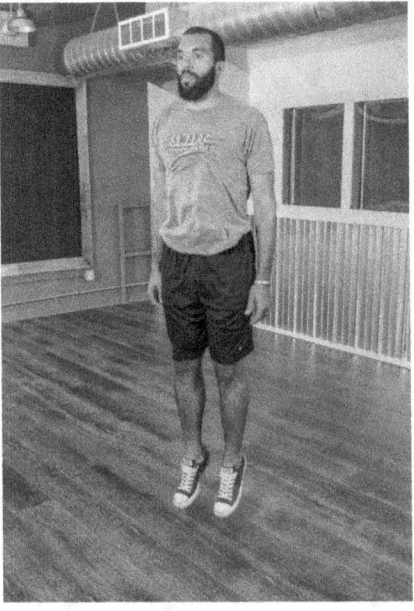

Jump up and down on the balls of the feet.

Jogging in Place on the Balls of the Feet

How to perform: Jog in place on the balls of your feet without letting the heels touch the ground.

Additional information: Absorb the landing on each foot and do not lock out the knees.

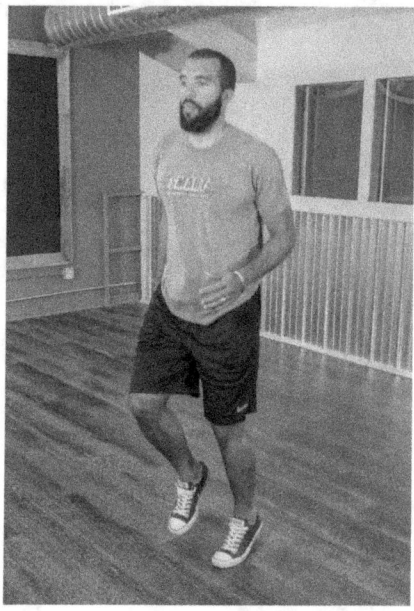

Run in place on the balls of your feet.

Mini Squat Jumps

How to perform: Stand feet shoulder-width apart and toes facing forward. Sit the butt back slightly loading the hips and lower body; then jump up extending through the feet, knees, and hips. Land softly with control by absorbing the ground through the feet, knees, and hips.

Additional information: Don't allow the knees to collapse inward or go forward past the toes throughout. When landing, land with the balls of the feet hitting first, followed by the rest of the feet and heels.

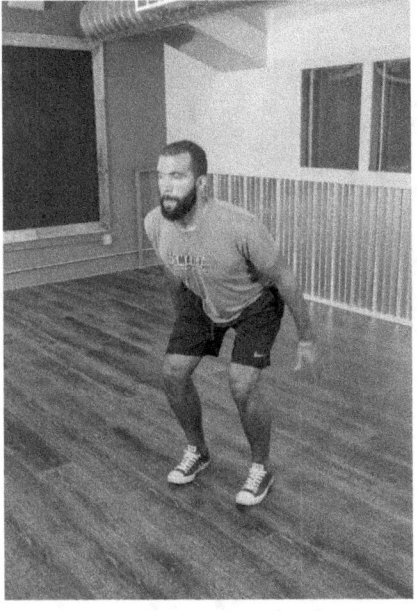

(a) Loading the hips and lower body preparing to jump;

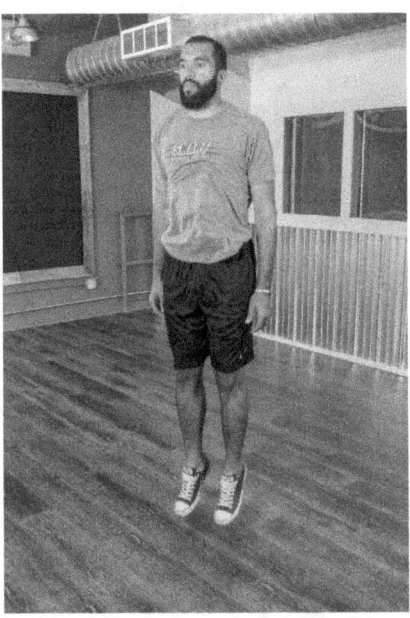

(b) Jumping up in the air.

Good mechanics Include:

— The knees do not collapse inward or go past the toes throughout.
— The hips are loaded prior to jumping and when landing.
— The landing is soft and controlled.

Single Leg Heel Tap

How to perform: Stand sideways at the edge of a step on one leg. Sit the butt back slightly and bend the stance knee, tapping the other heel to the floor. Stand back up, pushing the hips forward and squeezing the glut at the top.

Additional information: Keep the pelvis level. Do not allow the stance knee to collapse inward or go forward past the toes. You can hold on to a sturdy object for balance if needed.

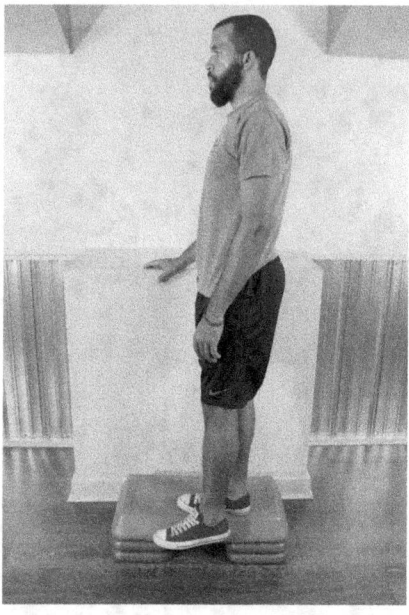 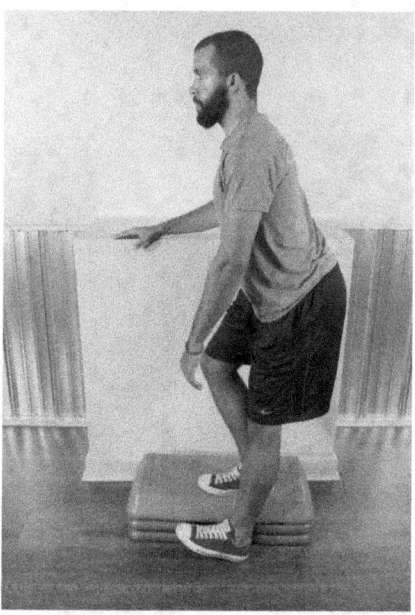

(a) Stand sideways on one leg at the edge of a step;

(b) Bend the knee and tap the heel to the floor.

How to Implement the SMART Performance® System

CREATING A PRACTICE PLAN

Use your individual results of the **SMART Performance®** system to create a practice plan. The foundational exercises, progressions, and the postural and upper body exercises will provide you with appropriate and effective exercises that you can do and build from to reach your health and fitness goals. Additionally, by following the foundational principals and criteria for running and jumping, you will have the ability and knowledge to choose safe fitness activities in the future.

For example, if your results showed ideal ability for all foundational, postural, and upper body exercises the exercises in your practice plan would be as follows (sample sets and reps included)

Exercise	Sets/Reps
Body weight squat	X20
Step back lunge	X20 Left and Right
RDL or SL RDL	X10 with 20 lb. or x10 Left and Right with 10 lb. in each hand
Push up	X20
Stability ball I,T,Y	X20 each with 5 lb.
Side lying ER or band ER	X20 Left and Right with 5 lb. or medium-tensioned band
Band IR	X20 Left and Right with medium-tensioned band
Scaption	X20 with 10 lb. in each hand
Overhead press	X20 with 10 lb.
Band row	X20 with medium-tensioned band
Single leg bridge	X20 Left and Right
Double leg lower	X20
Reverse ASLR	X20 alternating Right and Left
Plank	X1min hold
Side plank	X30sec hold Left and Right
Bird dog UE/LE	X10 Left and Right

The amount of sets, reps, and resistance can and should be varied depending on your ability level and fitness goals, but these initial exercises serve as a solid foundation. If an exercise is not appropriate for you to perform, you would simply substitute the appropriate progression and follow the system to progress. For example, if the sit-to-stand exercise was the most appropriate exercise for you initially, then you would perform that exercise and progress to learning the squat using the information in the **SMART Performance®** system.

USING MOBILITY AND STRETCHING:

The mobility and stretching section of the **SMART Performance®** system provides you with various stretches, mobility exercises, and tests for different areas of the body. If mobility is limited, use the appropriate stretches and mobility exercises to both improve motion and help progress foundational exercises that are affected. Regardless of your current mobility, the demands of life often create tightness and muscular imbalance. As a result, all individuals would benefit from performing stretching and mobility exercises on a regular basis to maintain good movement, flexibility, and help restore muscular balance.

An example of a complete stretching and mobility workout is as follows:

Exercise	Sets/Reps
Foam roll calf, HS, glut, quad, HF, ITB, T-spine	Focusing on tight areas
Hamstring wall or strap stretch	X1 min Left and Right
Straddle stretch	X1 min
Prone quad stretch	X1 min Left and Right
Half-kneeling hip flexor stretch	X1 min Left and Right
Pigeon or figure-4 glut stretch	X1 min Left and Right
Runners' stretch straight knee/bent knee	2X 30 sec Left and Right/ X10 Left and Right
Wall or stick shoulder flexion stretch	2X 30 sec Left and Right
Corner/doorway wall stretch or foam roll pec stretch	2X 30 sec
Sleeper stretch	2X 30 sec Left and Right
Foam roll T-spine extension	X10
Prone press up	X10
Prayer stretch, DKTC/SKTC, or seated flexion	X10

When choosing between stretches that focus on the same muscle areas or movements, choose the stretch that feels the best for you or creates the greatest improvement. Make sure you are able to relax during the stretch and focus on breathing. The hold times and reps given above for each exercise is a minimum, so take your time and don't rush the stretches. Use the foam roll exercises to normalize and maintain good soft tissue quality. If a muscle is knotted up, foam roll the muscle first before stretching it. Remember, for stretching to be effective, you have to feel a stretch but it should not be painful.

SMART Performance® Community

CONCLUSION

Congratulations! Learning to master the fundamentals of movement and exercise is a great start to achieving lasting physical health and wellness. I am confident that the content in this book will provide tremendous value and ensure a SMART start regardless of your fitness goals. But I also know people have different fitness goals and will have questions that were not specifically addressed in this book. As a result, I created the **SMART Performance®** Community. It is an online community designed to answer members' questions and help them gain a deeper understanding of the **SMART Performance®** concepts. Members will have access to supportive content, Q&A webinars, video lectures, community discussions, and newsletters. Additionally, I will provide specific content and answer questions about how to manage different types of muscle and joint pain. Go to www.smartperformanceconsultants.com today to join the **SMART Performance®** Community and continue working towards achieving your physical fitness goals.